Cancer
and the Search *for*
Lost Meaning

Cancer
and the Search *for*
Lost Meaning

The Discovery of a Revolutionary
New Cancer Treatment

Pier Mario Biava, MD

Foreword by Ervin Laszlo

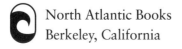

North Atlantic Books
Berkeley, California

Published by
North Atlantic Books
P.O. Box 12327   Cover and book design by Suzanne Albertson
Berkeley, California 94712   Printed in the United States of America

Cancer and the Search for Lost Meaning: The Discovery of a Revolutionary New Cancer Treatment is sponsored by the Society for the Study of Native Arts and Sciences, a nonprofit educational corporation whose goals are to develop an educational and cross-cultural perspective linking various scientific, social, and artistic fields; to nurture a holistic view of arts, sciences, humanities, and healing; and to publish and distribute literature on the relationship of mind, body, and nature.

North Atlantic Books' publications are available through most bookstores. For further information, call 800-733-3000 or visit our Web site at www. northatlanticbooks.com.

MEDICAL DISCLAIMER: The following information is intended for general information purposes only. Individuals should always see their health care provider before administering any suggestions made in this book. Any application of the material set forth in the following pages is at the reader's discretion and is his or her sole responsibility.

Library of Congress Cataloging-in-Publication Data

Biava, Pier Mario.
    Cancer and the search for lost meaning : the discovery of a revolutionary new cancer treatment / Pier Mario Biava ; foreword by Ervin Laszlo.
        p. ; cm.
    Summary: "Presents theories for curing cancer and bringing deeper meaning to peoples lives"—Provided by publisher.
        ISBN 978-1-55643-778-6
    1. Biava, Pier Mario. 2. Oncologists—Italy—Biography. 3. Cancer—Treatment—Research—Italy. 4. Cancer—Genetic aspects. I. Title.
        [DNLM: 1. Biava, Pier Mario. 2. Neoplasms—genetics—Personal Narratives. 3. Neoplasms—therapy—Personal Narratives. 4. Apoptosis—genetics—Personal Narratives. 5. Gene Therapy—trends—Personal Narratives. 6. Personal Satisfaction—Personal Narratives.
WZ 100 B5815b 2009]
RC265.8.B53A3 2009
616.99'4—dc22   2008036621

    1 2 3 4 5 6 7 8 9 UNITED 14 13 12 11 10 09

Contents

Foreword

This is without doubt one of the most remarkable books I have ever read. It is not like any other book—it is not one book, but three or more, integrated into a logical, organic unity. And all three contain essential information.

To begin with, this is the story of a personal insight that came unexpectedly and seemingly from out of the blue—an insight that holds the key to vanquishing one of the greatest scourges that has ever visited humankind: cancer. It is an account of the nature of that insight, of an "Einfall"—literally "falling in," as psychologists sometimes call it—an insight that provided the key to researching and developing an effective cancer cure. This book is also a treatise on the thinking that underlies this epochal discovery: a philosophical treatise that goes into the very foundations of our view of the world, and of life. And last but not least, this is a book of practical wisdom. It contains a well-founded criticism of the values and priorities that shape us and our world—a *"Zeitkritik"* in the classical and now ever more urgently needed sense. All three aspects of this multifaceted book have theoretical as well as practical significance.

In regard to the original Einfall, Dr. Biava's account is testimony that fundamental insights come to those who persistently and consistently seek solutions to the problems that occupy their mind, while remaining open to the intuitions that appear in their consciousness—and already in their subconscious. Biava's insight holds the key to solving the problem that scores of cancer researchers have been and are seeking: how to treat cells in the body that multiply without regard for the integrity of the rest. The classical way of dealing with this problem is to eliminate the malignant cells. The relevant insight here is that there is a softer and more effective way. Rather than excising or killing the malignant cells, they can be reprogrammed. With the right program they can transform into normal healthy cells, or else die off on their own accord.

The discovery of effective cellular re-programming, Dr. Biava argues, has not been, and very likely cannot be, made on the basis of the kind of thinking that dominates Western academic medicine. That kind of thinking is aimed at finding the formula for attacking and killing the malfunctioning cells and not at finding the way to re-program them. The latter approach derives from a different concept of the nature of the organism, and beyond that, of the nature of life. It is a systemic or, as it is popularly called, a holistic concept. Adopting it proves to be of great and immediate practical consequence. Among other things it provides a better understanding of malignancy in cells.

Dr. Biava's experience confirms Einstein's oft-cited pronouncement: one cannot solve a problem utilizing the kind of thinking with which the problem arose. In this instance it is not cancer itself that is the problem—for that is a state of the organism, a state found in the human body, as in other complex multicellular species. The problem to solve is how to *treat* this state: how to approach the body in which it arises. Biava's discovery is that malfunctioning cells need not always be excised, irradiated, or chemically destroyed: they can also be re-programmed for normal functioning. This is radically different thinking.

Even if the scalpel, chemotherapy, and irradiation are necessary in some cases, the effective treatment of cancer, Biava shows, is more subtle and more "soft" than that. It can consist of "convincing" the cells to re-program themselves to return to normal functioning—or to die off. This "convincing" is first of all metaphor, but it is close to the literal sense of the term, for it involves information, communication, and even a form of cognition. It will not be achieved, and not even attempted, so long as we regard the living organism as a biochemical mechanism where each cell is an individual entity with particular properties that can be tested and treated independently of the organic context in which it is found.

Yet the above is the dominant mistakenly reductionist concept. It holds sway in Western medicine, as well as in its offshoot, genetic engineering. It treats one particular cell, organ, or species of organism without regard to the effect of the treatment on the system of which that entity is a part. This is just as mistaken in regard to the health of the organism as it is in regard to the health of a society and the integrity of a bioregion's ecology. In society, for example, terrorists and other criminals are the functional equivalents of malignant cells. The mistaken "treatment" is to try to kill them and bombard the states and regions that harbor them. This seldom if ever works: in most cases the rogue individuals are replaced by others, and the "dis-ease" of society deepens. A better way would be to attempt to re-integrate the malfunctioning individuals and groups in a viable, integrally whole society.

Reductionism is the wrong way to try to heal any complex system, whether it is a community of cells or a community of humans. A cell, and a human being, is what it is mainly in the context of its relations to other cells and other individuals. The malignancy they may exhibit is contextual, and not individual-specific. As long as the context persists, malignant individuals will be generated in society, and malignant cells in the body. No part of a complex system is what it is in and by itself; it is what it is only in the context of its relations to the rest of the system.

The above insight is not new: it is the holistic concept classically expressed in the saying "the whole is more than the sum of the parts." More precisely, we should say that the whole provides the context that determines the nature and behavior of the parts. This is because the parts of a complex system are not related in a purely external, mechanistic way, as are the parts of a machine—parts that can be taken out, repaired, or replaced. Alfred North Whitehead called this kind of linkage "external relations." However, the relations of the parts in a living system are "internal." In internal relations, as Whitehead said, the part is what it is, functioning the way it functions, in accordance with its place and role within the whole.

The distinction between external and internal relations is not negligible. The assumption of external relations gives rise to reductionism in science, technology, as well as medicine. It underlies the conventional approach to cancer, and to scores of other diseases. Millions and indeed billions are spent on searching for solutions based on the reductionist philosophy of identifying, measuring, and then treating individual cells and organs. In so doing symptoms are often alleviated and battles are sometimes won. But the wars are mostly lost. The basic problems—the actual causes of the maladies—prove intractable.

In regard to the relation of parts to wholes, the reductionist philosophy misses the fact that there are two (not just one) kinds of causation. There is classical "upward causation" whereby the parts in interaction create the forces and produce the substances that act on the whole. In medicine this concept is applied by treating the part, in the belief that we can bring about health in the whole. This works in the case of relatively simple and straightforward malfunctions associated with specific organs and tissues. But in the complex case of cancer, where cells multiply regardless of the requirement of integrity in the body, it is too simplistic. Here we need to apply the concept of "downward causation" suggested by Nobel Laureate neurophysiologist Roger Sperry. In downward causation the whole exercises determinant influence on the parts. This kind of causation obtains in the brain and the higher nervous system where, as Sperry has shown, the consciousness exhibited by the whole brain determines the behavior of the brain's neuronal networks and subassemblies.

Alternative—or "complementary"—medicine goes beyond the reductionist stance of Western medicine: it attempts to treat the whole. Dr. Biava agrees that doing so through healthy lifestyles, a healthy environment, and healthy nourishment is an important factor, especially in preventing the occurrence of cancer, since the great majority of cancers are due to cellular mutations triggered by environmental factors. But once cancer has arisen, its actual treatment calls for a more fine-tuned approach. As Biava discovered, there is a way to make the whole organism "convince" its malignant cells to adopt the program of differentiation that makes them into healthy cells, or the program that leads to programmed cell death.

As the "programming" terminology suggests, the cure for cellular malignancy involves information, an important yet generally neglected element. Information exists not only when we speak, write, or otherwise communicate; it is present, and is indeed fundamental, in nature. A subtle and relatively recently discovered factor, it underlies the "entanglement" of particles and their "nonlocality" in the micro-domain. In the meso-domain of life, information underlies the coherence of the parts that constitute the organism, that is, the coherence of the whole organism. A high level of coherence is essential to the living organism: if it is not to succumb to the constraints of the physical world, its parts must be precisely yet flexibly correlated with each other. Without such correlation physical processes would break down the organization of the living state, bringing it closer to the inert state of thermal and chemical equilibrium. An organism is in thermal and chemical equilibrium only when it is dead. As long as it is living, it is in a state of *dynamic* equilibrium, and maintaining such equilibrium calls for fast and effective long-range correlations among its parts. Simple collisions among neighboring molecules—billiard-ball push-impact relations—must be complemented by a network of nearly instant communication that correlates all parts, even those that are distant from one another. Even rare molecules locate and respond to each other specifically, despite not being contiguous in the organism.

The presence of a high level of coherence throughout the organism suggests the presence of information in a distributed form. As

in a hologram, information is present in the living system simultaneously in all its parts; the parts are constantly and effectively "in-
formed" by the information that governs the whole. This is what
ensures the coordinated functioning of cells and organs; and it is
the lack of this that leads to the malfunctions that are manifested
as cellular malignancy.

In the last analysis cancer is a break in the flow of information
reaching given cells: it is a breakdown in communication between
the organism and some of its parts. Intra-organic communication
involves more than a mechanical transmission of signals: as Biava
points out, it is genuine communication, carrying meaning and presupposing some form of cognition.

How can a correct, health-sustaining flow of information be re-
established for malfunctioning cells? The answer to this question
is the substance of Biava's discovery. It is a complex answer that I
shall leave the reader to discover in the ensuing pages, but the basic
premise on which it rests is, like all insights of genius, remarkably
simple and logical.

Biava discovered that the information that "convinces" a malfunctioning cell to return to normalcy is produced by the living
organism, but it is produced only under specific circumstances.
Isolating the factors that carry this information and applying them
to malignant cells can re-program the cells and allow them to return
to normal functioning. The cell's program of *multiplication* changes
to a program of *differentiation*. This change obtains in the normal
course of development only in the embryonic stage, where the mother
"communicates" through her womb with the cells that compose
the fetus. This communication induces the stem cells to change at
the critical moment from multiplication to differentiation, thereby
beginning the process of organogenesis that leads to the fully developed fetus.

The essence of Biava's cure for cancer is to identify, extract, and
re-apply the information that stem cells receive in the mother's

womb to cancer cells in the fully developed organism. The information induces the cancer cells to shift from multiplication at the cost of damaging the integrity of the organism to differentiation and integration within the organism. In the case of certain varieties of cancer cell this proved possible. Further research is required to show whether it is possible in the case of other and perhaps all varieties of cancer cell.

There is more to bringing a discovery of this magnitude to the stage of practical application than elucidating the basic principle on which it rests. The "more" is painstaking work: persistent experimentation in the laboratory. It involves testing the alternatives that present themselves to see which of them work out. It means testing and testing, and testing again. There are more than a hundred different types of cancer cell, and each type responds to information in a specific way. What is information for one is merely insignificant noise for the other.

In the chapters of this book Dr. Biava recounts not only how he came by the key insight, but how he devoted years to testing and making it operational. This work is not completed yet, but the path to completing it is open. Now it is up to the science and medical communities to recognize that it is an open and effective path and to create the research networks to complete it. It is the earnest hope of this writer that the publication of this book will contribute to achieving this major goal. The vanquishing of cancer is in every human being's interest. The scourge of cancer is a sword of Damocles that hangs over the head of all.

Under the third aspect of this remarkable book, the aspect of *Zeitkritik*, I should note Biava's conclusions regarding the lessons that his work offers for human life and existence. The loss of meaning, he points out, is a principal characteristic of the modern age. Never before have human societies lacked meaning to such an extent. Cancer, Biava notes, is one of the by-products of this loss. It is a pathology of signification: the codes of healthy communication in the organism are negatively changed in tumor pathologies. Thus healing cancer is analogous to finding meaning in life. Both call for overcoming the fragmentation produced by mechanistically reductionist practices and technologies: for overcoming the fallacy of focusing on the part as if it were the seat of the malaise, instead of envisaging the whole web of relations in which the part is embedded. By shifting our sights from reductionism to systemic holism, we no longer attack the symptoms but can concentrate on treating the causes.

Before giving the floor to the author, one of the great minds and great benefactors of our time, I take the liberty of adding a personal note. Why did he, physician and medical researcher, turn to me, philosopher and systems theorist, to write a foreword to his book? And why did I agree to write it? The answer is the same to both questions. It turned out that, though we had very different starting points—Biava started from trying to find a cure to cancer, and I from trying to see what fundamental insights underlie current findings in the sciences—we reached basically the same conclusion. The world is not a mechanical aggregate of separate and separable parts, it is an organic unity, a nested hierarchy of wholes within wholes—of "holons," to use the term suggested by novelist-philosopher Arthur Koestler. Adopting the holistic worldview, far from being abstract theory, is of the greatest practical consequence. It makes all the difference in how we relate to each other in society, and how we deal with disease in our body. Health in us, and health around us, responds to the same basic insight: they are manifestations of the integrity and coherence of the systems that manifest it. Maintaining or recovering health calls for re-instating the flow of essential information in the systems. This is the way to heal the body, heal society, and heal the planet.

—*Ervin Laszlo*
New Year's 2008

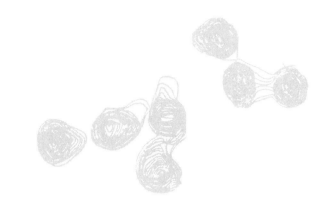

Chapter 1

Yellow-Orange

The sunsets in Trieste are beautiful, especially when the harsh Bora winds die down and the air is clear and electric, the sky blue and high. On days like these the bright and intense colors of the sunset are a wonderful sight to behold. The golden yellow of the sun turns into ochre and orange, then pale pink, dark red, and blends into shades of violet and purple and blue. The sun hides behind a single cloud whose white-gold lining gives off blades of bright yellow light that cut through the multi-colored layers of the sky. It's like looking at an immense Baroque painting that decorates the ceilings of certain churches and depicts God as a ray of light that from behind a cloud unleashes a blinding glare among a triumph of angels and colors.

The light, crisp air of Trieste is filled with sunlight during the day and intense colors at dusk. Seen from the coast on a clear, calm day Trieste looks like a city suspended in the air, wrapped in a streak of white that fades into the blue of the sea and the sky. Walking through the city on days like these, one is aware of a penetrating light that invades the streets and the piazzas, reaching even the narrowest and darkest alleyways. The light seems to make its way into your head and lungs, filling you with a sense of freedom and happiness that allows you to breathe more deeply and intensely.

One September evening on one of those beautiful days in Trieste I had left the hospital with an idea in my head that I couldn't get rid of. For three days I had thought of nothing else, living practically in a trance-like state, murmuring one-syllable answers to any questions I was asked. I was unable to communicate and this made me uneasy.

Mostly I was worried for my family, my wife, my children, who had been infinitely patient with me and had gotten used to seeing me at times completely engrossed in my thoughts. I am lucky to have a strong wife with a great sense of humor. When I would get lost in my thoughts, she would say to the kids, "Daddy is lost in the world of fairytales. Let's guess which fairytale he's imagining." When I came home absorbed in my thoughts, the kids would play with me and try to guess which fairytale I was lost in, and this would make me laugh and lift my spirits. I would joke around and make up stories, and our evenings became fun and light-hearted. This time, however, I had gone too far. I was unable to banish that idea from my head. I was fully aware of it, but I couldn't help myself.

As I left the hospital, the intense light that enveloped the city led me automatically toward the sea. I needed open space, I needed to breathe deeply and relax. Maybe this way I would be able to rest my mind and become more awake and in touch with reality.

That evening I resolved to reclaim my thoughts. A few abnormalities were acceptable, but this preoccupation was going too far. I refused to let this become a part of me. I had to stop the constant flow of thoughts that was overwhelming me and finally break free. Though not altogether clear in my mind, I think that was my intention as I made my way toward Audace Pier, which juts out into the gulf of Trieste.

The sunset was beautiful that evening, the light and colors bright. From the Carso Mountains the yellows, reds, and browns of autumn, together with the green grass and the white rock, became more intense. The sea, calm and blue, was speckled with gold, and a soft breeze lightly stirred the air. The boats were returning sleepily to the port, and old men were standing on the pier to watch the sunset, as was their custom. I raised my eyes to the sun and a glare of yellow-orange light suddenly blinded me, blotting out everything around me. In the intense brightness that surrounded me I suddenly saw exactly what I had been looking for. I perceived clearly what was at the basis of the biological processes that my mind had been lost in for the past three days looking for an answer, a solution. Finally the answer had arrived.

I was caught completely off guard. It was as if the solution had come from outside, from someone other than myself. For a moment I felt a sense of dismay and disorientation, but once I collected my bearings and strung together all the thoughts that for three days had run rampant in my mind, everything became clear. I understood what I had to do. My emotional tension suddenly disappeared and was replaced by a sense of quiet and well-being. That evening Trieste seemed even more beautiful. I was at peace with the world; I felt good, free, happy. I could finally go home.

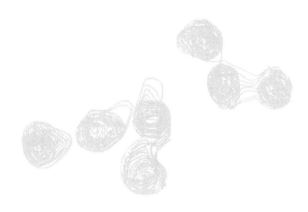

Chapter 2

A Flap of Butterfly Wings

From the time I decided to major in medicine, one thing was clear in my mind: I wanted to conduct scientific research, possibly in the field of oncology or diseases of the blood or immune system.

For this reason, from my early years as a student I had studied techniques of histology, those concerning the study of healthy and pathological bone marrow, those of *in vitro* cultures of normal and activated lymphocytes; and my further studies even included chromosomes and electronic microscope techniques. I studied pathological anatomy in depth, analyzing thousands and thousands of slides to visualize clearly in my mind the alterations due to the pathologies that I wished to further explore.

I was happy to study and learn new things. Doing research was fun and inspiring to me, and I found that my curiosity was continually being teased and fulfilled. After scrupulous preparation I was poised to pursue a scientific career. Yet suddenly, for reasons that are unclear to me, my choices and my life took a sharp turn in another direction.

I began to think that maybe research wasn't so important after all—that in fact to do it well, sufficient economic resources were enough, and that to some extent researchers were interchangeable. It was simply a question of organization and resources. The role of the individual was non-influential. After all, the major discoveries were the fruit of groups that worked in large state-of-the-art labs where individual creativity was sacrificed for structured work and study, with work plans devised by groups that received funding no doubt based on their scientific credibility, but also largely on their power. Therefore, I would have had to work in structured rather than creative groups and strive for power and scientific merit in areas of the community where merits are usually earned as a result of mainstream ideas instead of originality.

Having just finished medical school, it would be a long time before I could acquire either power or credibility. In the process I would grow old, my creativity would dwindle, and I would be left with only mediocre achievements. Given my lack of interest in credibility or power, I felt I was better off doing something else.

At that point, my career decisions were geared toward areas where I could establish human relations. I hoped to gain the opportunity to interact with interesting people who could inspire new and original ideas within me.

Essentially, my research activity did not involve so-called exact sciences but rather human sciences where, yes, organization and clout mattered, but less so. Indeed, I thought, unlike in biology, physics, chemistry or medical research, investments (even economic ones) within the context of human sciences did not exist. Choices within physical and biomedical sciences entailed decisions that gave enormous power to those who proposed and guided them. This would have had heavy consequences on the path taken, and the level of freedom in research could have been significantly limited by reasons that had nothing to do with the originality or importance of the research itself. I now realize as I write this that my decisions at the time were guided by devout individualism and were based on slightly simplistic reasoning. But there was nothing I could do about it. I was young and, like all youth, I was one-tracked and absolute. I did not have the luxury of drawing on the wisdom that comes with experience.

I finally decided to pursue the path of psychiatry, and my life changed dramatically. I say dramatic not only to mean the sense of subjective unease I felt as soon as I had made the decision, but also to convey in objective terms this turning point—a fork in the road, as it were—or radically different path I was on.

I figured that the second thoughts I had had on my role as a researcher were reason enough to throw away everything I achieved in six years and embark on an entirely new adventure. In this sense Edward Lorenz was absolutely right when in proposing mathematical models that could forecast meteorological events he described chaotic systems as being vulnerable to the "butterfly effect" whereby the flap of a butterfly's wings in Brazil can set off a tornado in Texas, and even the smallest changes in initial conditions can lead to dramatically different effects.[1]

Chaos had taken over my life and I was helpless in its wake, completely unprepared and lacking the basic skills to stay afloat. The change in my career path was enough to turn everything upside down. I was experiencing the butterfly effect of chaotic systems first-hand.

What upset me the most was that my wife would also be touched by the butterfly effect. I was married at this point and wanted a serene and happy home life, but the choice I was about to make would jeopardize any sense of security I had achieved. I had been offered a stable job as an assistant professor at the University of Pavia researching pediatric immunology, which I turned down in favor of this decision, a decision that meant giving up prospects for a secure job and moving city to city on unstable terrain. Fortunately, my wife loves adventure and has always supported me in my explorations into unknown territories. Her support and enthusiasm have always been crucial to my accomplishments.

As a psychiatrist I had stubbornly taken the toughest route by choosing to work in the most difficult sectors in the first ever mental health centers opened in Italy in those years.

These centers had been created based on Franco Basaglia's experience with psychiatric hospitals, and at the time these health centers were simply a territorial extension of mental institutions. However, in the city of Reggio Emilia these centers had been set up by the regional government as an alternative to psychiatric hospitals. The regional officials and hospitals agreed on a policy whereby the hospitals would encourage patients with less serious illnesses and who were sufficiently autonomous to leave the hospital.

These patients would then be looked after in their homes by a team headed by a different (not affiliated with the hospital) technical-scientific and organizational director. In addition, the regional government provided financial assistance to these patients so that they could live at home. In other words, these centers were the first alternative to hospitalization and an attempt to render psychiatric assistance more civil, humane, and modern.

The demission policy turned out to be a disaster. The teams were faced with extremely difficult cases. I personally went from town to town all along the Po Valley and up into backwaters of the Apennine Mountains in the areas of Reggio Emilia and Modena. These people lived in remote places and suffered terrible visual and audio hallucinations.

One of these patients was named Zita. She lived in a dark corner in her wooden house in a small mountain village with a population of no more than twenty, making any real human interaction virtually impossible. She would scream that she saw and heard violent monsters. When I visited her she would gradually calm down and tell me about her nightmares and her fears. Our meetings seemed to help her. She would walk me out to the car and during the winter months if there was snow she would stop to pick up a fistful and eat it like a little girl.

I also recall Andrea. He was in his thirties and had been abandoned in a nursing home for the elderly. When I went to see him the head of the facility warned me to be careful because Andrea was a dangerous paranoiac. In fact, he was the most harmless person in the world. To survive the hurtful events that had scarred him and to avoid actually killing himself, Andrea had decided, in an extreme process of sublimation and rationalization, that he was dead. It was no small task convincing him that he was not dead and that in fact he still had a good chance to re-connect with life thanks to the support my colleagues and I would give him. Andrea returned to his home in a small village in the mountains near Modena, and for a long time we made daily visits and slowly his rebirth began. Then things took a turn for the worse. We had too many patients to look after and they were all difficult cases. There simply was not enough time to look after them properly. Without our strong support Andrea was unable to make it—he "died" again and was sent back to the nursing home.

These setbacks were very difficult for me to deal with. Personnel and facilities were sorely lacking; we could only rely on our private offices. There were no structured facilities or possibilities for short hospital stays. The only resources we had access to were our own therapeutic abilities.

This was truly the dawn of a reform that later would be extended to the rest of Italy. My colleagues who were older and more experienced than I had the defense mechanisms to endure the stress of such a challenging job. Not only was I too young, but inside I still felt a longing for those years I spent as a researcher. I knew I wouldn't last long with the regret I felt inside and with such a terribly difficult job. I admired my colleagues, and remembering them now I still feel the same admiration. However, it was absurd for me to continue down that road and betray my desires, interests, and true nature. I had to admit that one's own nature cannot be denied. I had to remedy the mistakes I had committed.

What's more, there was no intellectual satisfaction from that type of work since the study of psycho-social dynamics that resulted in a specific state of psychic illness were nearly always so clear and evident in their cruelty that no particularly in-depth analyses were necessary.

The real problem lay in the prevention of psychotic disorders. So, with the support of Mental Health Services, I began meeting with various workers in different industries throughout the area to tackle the issue of what could be at the root of their psychological problems. The union organizations and the regional government whose goal it was to provide occupational medical services to the industrial workers supported these meetings.

I soon realized that the workers knew pretty much what was causing their psychological problems, and that I was much happier in this role. This latter was due to two reasons: first, the work I was doing was in fact innovative research that stimulated my curiosity and piqued my interest. Second, I was better able to handle the situations with which I was confronted since I was not alone in tackling insurmountable problems. I felt the support and involvement of the workers, and together we searched for common solutions.

When the regional government organized the occupational medical services (the first in Italy to be directly managed by a regional authority) and asked me to act as its Director, I accepted. Occupational medicine gave me the chance to conduct research in fields and sectors that were much wider than those inherent to the study of psychic disorders alone.

The areas of research were limitless, from risks linked to the different production processes and the related pathologies, to the evolution of technological cycles and of research methods for industrial health and toxicology, to issues associated with industrial environmental pollution. Early on my objective in the field of occupational medicine became clear to me. I wanted to study the relationship between man and environment and research the links between disease and environmental risk factors. This was my chance to address issues that were relevant and had a strong impact on human health. I wouldn't be limited to basic research but would be involved in applied research. When I had graduated from medical school this wasn't exactly what I envisioned myself doing, but perhaps this type of research would lead to immediate and concrete results that would help reduce health risks for specific groups of workers. This was enough to satisfy me. If I also considered that in those years the battles being waged by the unions for the health of factory workers constituted a highly innovative research project to change the risk conditions in the workplace—a goal that involved the workers directly taking part in the project—then I could consider myself completely gratified.

During my first years in Reggio Emilia I intensely researched the ceramics sector, which was the main industry in the area of Scandiano-Sassuolo. A clear cause-and-effect link emerged from my research on environmental risks and the health condition of workers. Unfortunately, in those years research showed that many workers had lead poisoning and silicosis, as well as various other pathologies linked to their use of dyes and colorings and exposure to other risks.

Although my research activities had been fruitful, I was forced to admit that because of the political situation at that time the involvement of the unions in the research had become excessively invasive and was jeopardizing the autonomy of the technicians. The strategy of the unions aimed to obtain greater contractual power in the work environment; consequently medical and technical analyses became of marginal interest to them. In fact, research, particularly long-term research, was often seen as an obstacle to the union's contractual ends. At that point it was clear that the interests of the unions and those of the physicians and technicians had diverged. I tried several times to convince the union representatives that their stance was damaging to the physicians and certainly would not lead to any changes in medicine, a goal which they claimed they sought to achieve. Obviously, the restrictions we faced hindered our medical practice. On their part the regional government officials had absolutely no interest in curbing the invasiveness of the unions.

There were never-ending discussions with public representatives and the workers' representatives as to what relationships the political-union organizations would have with the healthcare professionals, but no adequate solution was ever reached. I deemed that the only way to force the parties to face up to their responsibilities was to tender my resignation to the regional government authorities.

In the meantime, I had finished my specialization in Padua, where I met a professor who was well-versed in numerous fields of industrial medicine. The professor had moved from Padua to Trieste, where he was employed by the university. He offered me a position as assistant professor, and I was more than happy to accept. I was finally free to study the problems that were presented to me from time to time. Furthermore, I was confident that with the guidance of a good teacher I would become a good doctor.

I arrived in Trieste and immediately felt disoriented. No doubt the city was beautiful, but it seemed foreign. It didn't feel like I was in Italy, but rather in a city in Central Europe and in certain instances almost in the Orient. The atmosphere was relaxed and very retro. The city seemed to move in slow motion and flow like the placid waves of the calm sea that wets its shores. Time seemed to stand still. This appealed to me a great deal because it reminded me of my childhood, when the slow movement of time created space for dreaming and imagining.

Perhaps its unusual, almost dream-like atmosphere was the reason Trieste was a cradle for great literature. The cocoon-like environment did wonders to ease the tension I had accumulated in Reggio Emilia and erased it for good. It's no surprise that the leitmotiv of the way of life in Trieste that I quickly learned is to *viva la' e po bon* or "take life as it comes" because that is exactly how life is lived there.

This fatalism characterizes the spirit of the people of Trieste and their philosophy on life. I soon forged friendships with my young colleagues, and together we frequented the city's local restaurants and *osmizze*[2] in the Carso Mountains, singing songs and causing a ruckus. On one of our first nights out they made me face a reality of existence that one usually tries not to think about. They took a meter stick and placed it on a sheet of paper and instructed me to put a mark at 72 and 28, which was my age at the time. Although

I was still young, actually seeing the distance that separated my age from the average age at which males die (the average age has since increased for both men and women) really made me stop and think. You realize that life must be lived to the fullest and that you must be in tune with the present, being aware of every second and at peace with yourself and others. This Epicurean and fatalist vision deeply characterizes the people of Trieste and is immediately palpable, along with the melancholy that lies at the heart of this. Life is brief and fleeting as time inexorably passes by. Herein lies the irresistible allure of the city that strikes you even more than its beauty and marks you deeply.

I encountered this philosophy on life also during my work at the hospital. I worked several night shifts and had come face to face with death. Patients whose life was slipping away from them would often refuse my stubborn attempts to save them and tell me: "Doctor, you've done enough. I'm old and have lived as much as I can. Go and have fun and don't worry about me." That's exactly what they would say: "Go and have fun." Being faced with such a profound and natural acceptance of existence, even of death, left me shocked and confused. This vision of life was adopted by the elderly and young alike.

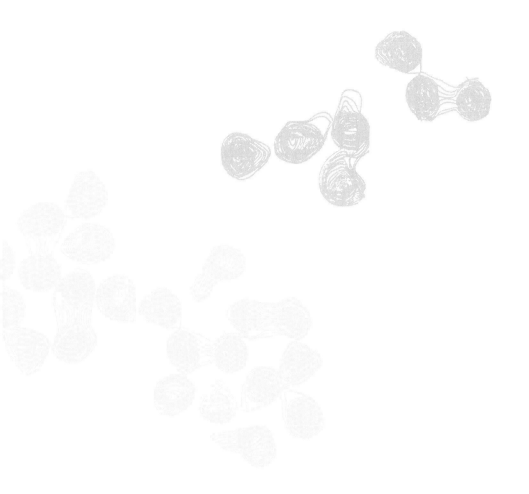

Chapter 3

A Strange Attractor

My work within the Occupational Health Institute at the University of Trieste enabled me to come into contact with a great variety of people and problems. Since the Institute was within the Riuniti Hospital of Trieste and had hospital beds, patients with recognized diseases as well as those with other pathologies were hospitalized and treated there. The doctors of the Institute were not only responsible for treating the patients that were hospitalized in their ward, they also had to take on day and night shifts as internal physicians for all the other wards. Besides general medicine, the doctors obviously had to deal with the wide range of problems relating to occupational medicine, not only diagnosing professional diseases, but especially preventing them. Indeed, most of the medical activity was carried out directly at work sites where the doctors conducted environmental and epidemiological investigations. Therefore, the work I did in Trieste was very complex and interesting, which is why I liked it so much, even though it was often very tiring, especially when I was on the night shift at the Maggiore Hospital in Trieste (which is the main unit of the Riuniti Hospital).

I will never forget my first New Year's Eve in Trieste. I was on duty at the hospital and was a little worried because in the meantime my wife had been hospitalized while pregnant with our second child. She was past her due date and I was concerned. The night shift of the Maggiore Hospital in Trieste was especially difficult. For twelve hundred beds there was only one internist on duty, together with one surgeon, a cardiologist, and an intensive care physician. The first to be called was the internist (as an industrial physician, I acted as an internist) who, if necessary, would then alert one of the other physicians. At that time, and maybe even now, the population of Trieste was one of the oldest in Italy. Most of the hospital's patients were elderly and suffered from serious pathologies. On average, five or six people would die every night. I remember that just before midnight on this New Year's Eve, an elderly man died. In these cases the hospital notifies the patient's relatives to come to the hospital as quickly as possible.

A few minutes before midnight all the hospital staff had gathered to ring in the New Year. I went down to join them, and at the stroke of midnight we raised our glasses for a toast. At that same instant the dead patient's son walked in. I was clearly embarrassed and asked my colleagues to put off the toast. I gave the son the news of his father's death and explained the causes that had led to his dying. As soon as I had finished talking someone offered him a glass, he took it, and to my surprise and unease he said, "Doctor, what can you do? My father is dead and there's nothing we can do to change that. I loved him very much and I remember all the good and bad times we had together. Life goes on and we have to go on with it."

I felt as if I had landed on another planet. In Lombardy, we're more inclined to keep up appearances, so I was shocked by his bluntness. Ever since then I've tried to take life as it comes and ride its waves and storms.

As an industrial physician at the hospital I conducted clinical treatment activity and applied research. One of the first studies I carried out in Trieste was on pathologies arising from asbestos. I knew from the literature that in seaport cities, where there is a well-developed naval-mechanical industry, the incidence of malignant pleural mesothelioma, a rare tumor, was quite high. This was due to exposure to asbestos, which in the shipyards was often used to insulate pipes and boilers and to build bulkheads, among other things. In the areas where the ships were built, and especially where they were repaired, pipes and walls were ripped out and demolished, making exposure to asbestos especially high.

Analyzing the statistics on work accidents and illnesses, I found that not a single case of work-related pleural mesothelioma had been reported at that time in Trieste. This seemed very strange to me. I figured that this could have been due to the lack of knowledge on this pathology and the related risks. To verify this hypothesis, I examined the archives of the Riuniti Hospital in Trieste. All the chest X-rays that could be meaningful for this pathology were selected. Obviously, for a diagnosis both the anatomic and histological reports were necessary.

From this point of view, a practice that was unique to Trieste out of all the Italian cities was pivotal to my study. Essentially, unlike other Italian cities, where terminal patients are returned home, in Trieste if a person at home was gravely ill, he or she would be taken to the hospital. Consequently, almost the entire population of Trieste died in the hospital. On top of this, Trieste had an extremely efficient pathological anatomy ward that performed autopsies on all the people who died in the hospital. In short, almost one hundred percent of the people who died in Trieste were autopsied. This way it was possible to study the cases of death that were recorded and have a clear picture of the trends of the various pathologies affecting the population.

This inexhaustible source of information, however, also gave rise to general risks and caused high levels of stress among the physicians and medical staff. I remember enduring very high stress, especially during the night shifts.

There was a professor in the pathological anatomy ward who was, shall I say, very dedicated to his job and would arrive at five o'clock every blessed morning, including Sunday. He would start calling all the wards to learn the number of deceased. The procedure was to transport the deceased to the morgue so that around nine o'clock they could all be autopsied. During the night shift the physician had to fill out the death certificate, which I refused to do so soon after death had been pronounced. I would visit the deceased several times to ensure that he or she was in fact dead, and only around eight o'clock when I ended my shift and was certain of death would I fill out the certificate.

Despite all these precautions, sometimes the stress would play tricks, even on the nursing staff. I recall one morning a patient in my ward had been transferred to surgery, and another patient had died during the night. The respective case sheets had to be sent to the respective wards. At one point surgery called asking for our patient's file, the patient who had to undergo surgery. The nurse answering the phone replied that the file had already been sent down. But the surgery ward had received the file bearing the name of the dead patient to be transferred to the morgue. At this point the nurse began to panic and lose all ability to think. Out of breath, she called the morgue and asked if the patient who was supposed to undergo surgery was there. The name was indeed the same. She instructed them to stop immediately and not perform the autopsy. But the autopsy had already been performed. The nurse fainted right then and there. A simple file mix-up had been enough to provoke this abnormal reaction, a clear sign of the level of stress that these situations entailed.

Although the activity of the pathological anatomy ward posed many problems, I have to say that the amount of data available from the ward had been useful on several occasions. In my experience it no doubt had been. After identifying the cases with a radiological history of suspect pleural mesothelioma, the histological report and autopsy report were examined. They confirmed the diagnosis in more than a hundred cases, making Trieste one of the cities in Italy with the highest incidence of the pathology. In addition, reconstructing the work history of the deceased through interviews with relatives confirmed exposure to asbestos in more than eighty percent of the cases, thereby revealing a causal link (the relative risk was extremely high) between exposure and disease.

The publication of this data led the unions to take action. They signed an employment agreement with shipyard officials and the

Port Authority of Trieste where asbestos arrived in large quantities in burlap sacks that were ineffective in preventing the particles from being released into the air. Thanks to this agreement, asbestos was banned in workplaces and replaced by more suitable materials. As a result, asbestos risks were eliminated in Trieste about fifteen years earlier than in the rest of Italy.

Regretfully, although asbestos was eliminated in those years, it was predictable that deaths due to pleural mesothelioma would continue in the areas of Trieste and Monfalcone, where asbestos was widely used in the shipyards. The scientific works that we published following the research predicted that deaths by pleural mesothelioma would continue to occur for a long time. Unfortunately, our predictions were correct. In the area of Trieste and Gorizia, people continue to die due to asbestos even many years after exposure. This is because the latency period from the beginning of exposure to the clinical manifestation of the tumor is very long and in the case of asbestos can reach up to forty years. The deaths recorded today in Trieste and Gorizia are caused by exposure to asbestos that occurred in the 1970s or 1980s.

My research on pleural mesothelioma inspired me to delve deeper into the problems arising from exposure to environmental carcinogens. I started to conduct a series of research projects on chemical carcinogens in many companies, in particular in the tanneries around Udine. There, in addition to the chromium utilized in the tanning process, many other cancer-causing dyes were used. This research also led me to analyze in depth the theoretical and experimental aspects of environmental carcinogens. I collected much of the literature available at the time on the subject with the help of a professor whom I knew well and who was the director of the International Agency for Research on Cancer of Lyon (IARC). He sent me all the monographs published by the Agency on environmental carcinogens, and thus I began my systematic study. I realized that the problems related to environmental carcinogens could not be separated from those stemming from exposure to substances or agents that caused DNA cellular mutations (mutagens) and embryonic malformations (teratogens).

My studies on the relationship between carcinogens and agents that give rise to mutations or malformations focused on data from literature that evidenced how carcinogenic agents administrated during pregnancy in laboratory animals had different effects depending on the period in which they acted. The number of malformations or miscarriages rose if the agent was administrated during the period in which the organs and systems of the embryo are formed (organogenesis); and tumors in the offspring arose when the agents acted in the period during which the formation of organs and systems was complete. Why did this occur? Why during organogenesis did the mutation of the genoma—which usually constitutes the start of carcinogenesis—express itself as a malformation or a miscarriage, but not as a malign transformation of the cells? What causes malformed tissue to be created during organogenesis despite the fact that it is made up of differentiated cells and not of cells that multiply continuously and indefinitely like tumor cells? What causes the spontaneous death of the embryonic cells (miscarriage) and inhibits the formation of a tumor?

These were the questions that flashed through my mind, held it prisoner and forced me into a three-day-long condition in which I nearly lost contact with reality and was trapped in an almost hallucinatory state where my thoughts scrambled for a solution.

At last, the solution came to me that evening at sunset on the pier in Trieste. What I had seen was an action mechanism that prohibits cells from becoming cancerous, even if they are exposed to the action of a carcinogen. In practice, I had visualized the correction system that the embryo uses to defend itself from genetic damage. In the yellow-orange light that blinded me I saw a molecule of a carcinogen cause mutations in the DNA and another molecule immediately correct it. These corrections therefore allowed the cell to differentiate and not remain trapped in its maturing process. The lack of differentiation consequent to the mutation had to be the core of the process. The mutation was not enough; the differentiation process had to be stopped to cause cancer.

From this perspective, the tumor cell was an undifferentiated cell, mutated and trapped in a stage of multiplication between two phases of differentiation. In other words, the tumor cell had to be mutated and almost certainly have grave alterations to its genetic expression with an imbalance of the genoma toward an embryonic configuration. The tumor cells therefore had to be very similar to stem cells at a different degree of differentiation. However, unlike these latter, which can develop and differentiate completely, the tumor cells could not complete their development to fully mature cells due to the mutation they had undergone. This mutation had separated the programs of differentiation and multiplication.

After I had mentally visualized this process and recovered from the shock, I immediately understood what was happening in the processes leading to malformations or miscarriages.

In these cases, the mutations are not completely corrected, thus giving rise to malformations that may be life-compatible or, if the insult to the DNA is too severe, may kill the embryonic cells (miscarriage). In any case, the malformations and miscarriages are the final result of a genetic insult that occurs during organogenesis. During the time when life is being created, cancer formation is inhibited. Rather than allow the formation of a tumor, the embryo's system of correction and control kills off all the embryonic cells, thus resulting in a miscarriage. At most, the system will allow life-compatible mutations. In this case, altered tissue made up of differentiated cells is allowed to form. However, when organogenesis is completed and all the organs have been formed, the system of correction and control of cell differentiation becomes less efficient. Moreover, unlike the embryo, the fetus (so-called when the embryo's organogenesis has been completed) no longer possesses a regulatory system that is able to repress the multiplication genes activated by the cancer genesis process and trigger the cell differentiation process. In this instance, the administration of carcinogenic agents causes cancer in the offspring.

Finally, it was clear what I had to do. I had to verify through experimentation if the factors that are present in the different stages of stem-cell differentiation were able to re-differentiate cancer cells by bypassing the mutations that are at the origin of the malignity. These factors are present only once in a lifetime—i.e., when life is being formed in the embryonic stage—and are no longer present in the fetus, at least not in a significant amount. I had to face the task of probing the embryo to identify the different stages of differentiation and therefore locate these factors.

At the time, in the 1980s, stem-cell research was by no means practiced like it is today and very little was known about it. I could rely on limited scientific references. Strangely, however, I quickly realized that I was tackling a matter of biology, which for quite a while had interested me but which I had pushed aside. In fact, during the final years of my university studies I had set up a course at the Borromeo College in Pavia managed by the Institute of Genetics and Molecular Biology of the University of Pavia precisely on cellular differentiation and stem cells. As for the stem cells of hematopoietic tissue, I had studied chromosomal maps during my time at medical school. Now, years later, I was at a crucial point of an issue of biology that had intrigued me since I was a student. So, even though I had done everything I could to avoid purely basic research, in the end I found myself dealing with exactly the subject that I had always wanted to examine further.

I had taken the path of chaos, but in the end I realized that chaos acts with an implacable determinism. Chaos had brought me right to my starting point. After so much zigzagging, a strange attractor had led me home. Perhaps behind chaos and its strange attractors lies something else, which some call destiny or fate, while others call it Providence or Karma. In any event, our origin and that of life and everything in the world involves a series of chaotic events that in the end reflects an incredible level of order. The term "attractor" in chaos theory only represents our ignorance in interpreting and explaining the order that, with infinite intelligence, is established at the edge of chaos.

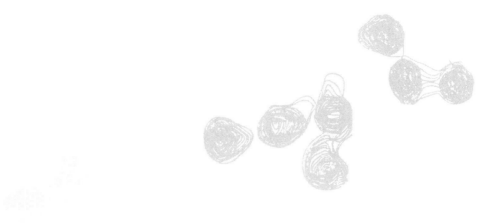

Chapter 4

The Castle in the Carso Mountains

U nfortunately, the Occupational Health Institute could not offer me the resources I needed to conduct my research. Its activity was limited to studying the level of physical and chemical agents that workers were exposed to and quantifying the effects; it was not equipped to conduct research on *in vitro* cell cultures or lab animals.

My aim was to research cancer cell cultures *in vitro*, but in the early 1980s there were no local institutes at university level that conducted studies of this kind. I was therefore forced to turn my attention to lab animals. I wasn't exactly thrilled about this decision because it went against my ecologist convictions, but at the time it was the only way to conduct experimental research in the field of oncology in Trieste. Setting up a facility for *in vitro* research, training personnel, and obtaining the necessary instruments would have been a lengthy and costly process, and I wasn't even sure if it was worth it since I had no way of predicting whether or not my idea would be confirmed. What if it wasn't? What would I have done with an *in vitro* research lab considering that my institute conducted mostly applied research? I decided to perform my first experiment on lab animals to find out if my intuition had been correct.

I promised myself that I would only perform initial tests. If the validity of my research was unconfirmed then I would stop there, but if it was confirmed then I would no longer use lab animals and I would organize my research some other way.

My curiosity to find out whether or not my idea could be verified led me to contact my colleagues at the Institute of Pharmacology, where they had a laboratory animal facility in which they performed several experiments, mostly on the efficacy of chemotherapeutic drugs. The Institute was located in a rather unusual building.

Essentially, it was a small castle with a tower, located near the new Fascist-era university.

To reach the castle you had to take a main road to the Opicina area in the Carso Mountains, turn onto a narrower road toward the main building of the campus, go up a steep mountain road and pass through the woods. Traveling along a precipice protected by a low wall, you come to an opening where you can enjoy a wonderful view of the entire gulf of Trieste. There sits the castle.

The original exterior of the castle had been preserved, with mullioned windows, arched doorways, and battlements along the top of the castle walls. Inside, it had been completely renovated and transformed into a series of modern labs that were clean and comfortable. Overall, the atmosphere was pleasant and luminous. From the windows you could look out onto the city and see the wide expanse of green of the mountains and the blue sea.

The pharmacologists who worked there were very nice to me and listened carefully to my plan, reassuring me that I could use their facility and equipment and work there whenever I pleased. There was just one hitch: I had to find funding for the research since all their money had been allocated to projects that were already underway and that they obviously could not interrupt. I was perfectly fine with this. All I had to do was find financial support for my research.

The Occupational Health Institute had a small budget set aside for research projects. The money was provided by the university. However, the fund was reserved for occupational health studies and could not be used for the purposes I had in mind. I could have asked for a grant from the Italian Research Council, but unfortunately by that time the deadline for filing the request for funding had expired, and I had no intention of letting another year go by to wait for another competition. Besides, if they accepted my project I could start only after two or three years, an eternity for me at that time.

But luck was on my side. My brother-in-law contacted me. He

and I had studied together in high school and college and ended up marrying two sisters within a short time of each other. Destiny had kept us apart and now had brought us together. He had become the Managing Director in Europe of an American multinational pharmaceutical company that was organizing a multi-centric study on a low-dose single administration of antibiotics. Since he knew I worked in a diagnostic and therapy ward, he asked me if I wanted to take part in the study. It had never occurred to me that I could work on behalf of a pharmaceutical company. It was at that moment that I understood that this job might give me the opportunity to secure the funds I needed to conduct my research.

In those years, regulations on university-level clinical research stipulated that the pharmaceutical industry incur research costs and allocate sums, as agreed from time to time, to the university, the hospital, and the researchers. I asked my brother-in-law if I could use my share to purchase lab mice. He thought my request was a bit strange, but since financially it would make no difference to the company, he agreed.

Since I believed that the mechanism at the root of slowing tumor growth was based on the regulation of gene cell multiplication and differentiation, I decided to conduct my experiments on syngeneic, or genetically identical, mice in order to avoid an immune response due to the exchange of protein molecules between two mice. In this way, any positive results could not be attributed to an immune response.

For the experiment the mice had to be impregnated, and the embryo had to be isolated at the start of gastrulation—in other words, during the stage in which embryo stem cells start to differentiate—and the factors present in that stage had to be extracted and injected in the mice in which a tumor had been implanted. Isolating the embryo from the pregnant uterine mucous membrane was much trickier than I expected. At the stage when the embryo is extracted it is some hundreds of micrometers in size (one thousandth of a millimeter), but this problem was easily solved by using a stereomicroscope. The biggest problem was due to the fact that at that stage the embryo is deeply nestled into the pregnant uterine mucous membrane, so it is difficult to completely extract tiny fragments of mucus so strongly attached to the surface of the embryo. Even though I was using a stereomicroscope, through which it was possible to clearly see the entire embryo and its contours, I still was not sure that all residual pregnant uterine mucous membrane had been extracted from the embryo. We wanted to be certain that we were using only tissue from the embryo and that not even the tiniest fragment of uterine mucous tissue could contaminate the experiment. Therefore, the experiment was conducted not only on the group of mice treated with differentiated embryonic factors and a control group (not treated), but also on a group treated with factors extracted from the pregnant uterine mucous membrane and a group treated with factors extracted from non-pregnant uterine mucous membrane. Finally, to avoid any aspecific effects due to the administration of biological products, I decided to also test a hepatic extract from another group of mice.

Making different groupings turned out to be a good move on my part. The first experiment showed dramatic effects, not in the group treated with differentiated embryonic factors, but in the group treated with factors extracted from the pregnant uterine mucous membrane.

In this group, all the mice survived and were free of cancer, while in all the other groups the mice died with widespread pulmonary metastasis. The results took me by surprise and I was happy that something, something truly exciting, had happened.

At this point, I decided to repeat the experiment and personally monitor the results. The first thought that entered my mind was that an exchange had taken place in the identification of the mice groups. I had to monitor the entire process, including the management of the groups in the laboratory animal facility, and so the experiment was repeated.

Every morning I would walk from my house to the research lab, about a mile away. This was one of the best times of my life. It was spring, with the trees sprouting their first leaves and the flowers beginning to bloom. During my walks I would come across peach trees and newly budded wild rose bushes. Before reaching the castle, as I made my way through the woods, I would encounter squirrels and deer. Except for the portion of my walk where I had to cross the main road, my treks were surrounded by a profound silence. The air was cool and electric. The nice weather held out for the entire month-long duration of the experiment. The sky was high and bright blue, typical of Trieste on nice days. As I walked, I grew excited in anticipation for the outcome of my experiments.

Before the experiments were concluded I realized that the results were the same as the previous ones: the healthy mice group was the one treated with the factors extracted from the pregnant uterine mucous membrane. At the end of the experiment, that was the only group that survived. All the other groups died of large primary tumors and pulmonary metastasis. At this juncture, I began thinking that the problem of cell development and differentiation in the embryo in mammals was much more complex than was believed, and that the maternal uterus was not merely a mechanical container but rather a regulating organ.

If you think about it, this explains why mammal embryos develop in the mother's uterus, where the unfolding of the new life can be controlled. Maybe, I thought, the mother's uterus is an organ that through evolution serves to protect the life and ensure the survival of the embryo, unlike ovoviviparous animals. Certain substances vital to the development and differentiation of the embryo are contained in the mother's womb, and these play an important role in the protection against cancer.

These considerations led me to think about using embryos of

ovoviviparous animals, which already contain all the information for differentiation and complete development.

Again, luck was on my side. Just before reaching the castle, in the middle of the woods, there is a modern, one-story glass building well integrated into the landscape. It is the Institute of Zoology. A professor and friend of mine worked there and was studying the development of embryos of *Drosophila melanogaster,* the fruit fly.

Now, in evolutionary terms this animal is very far from a mouse, and its genes and proteins are in part different. However, some part had to be similar, and it was likely that much of the differentiation factors would be maintained during phylogenesis (evolution) and that therefore they would be the same. So I decided to use Drosophila embryos for my next experiment.

I couldn't expect a dramatic outcome with the complete arrest of cancer formation, as occurred in the previous experiments in which I used substances extracted from the pregnant uterine mucous membrane of mammals, but if the original idea had been correct and if the differentiation factors were maintained during phylogenesis, at least some effect would be observed. I asked my friend to give me some Drosophila embryos at the blastoderma stage (the stage in which embryo stem cells start to differentiate).

Extracting and using differentiation factors of Drosophila was infinitely less complicated than with the mice. The experiments were easy to conduct and interpret. The statistical analyses revealed that compared to the control group, the development of the primary tumor had slowed down significantly and the survival time had doubled in the treated group.

From this I concluded that in the stage in which embryos start to differentiate it is possible to obtain factors that are able to inhibit or slow down tumor growth. These factors are directly present in the embryos of ovoviviparous animals, which contain all the information for complete development, while in mammals these factors are also found in the maternal uterus, a regulatory organ.

At this point, two paths lay before me and I intended to pursue them both. My goal was to clarify the various complex aspects that the earlier experiments revealed. I had to ascertain whether the isolated substances gave rise to not just one type but different types of cancer, including human cancer. I had to examine what mechanisms were responsible for slowing tumor growth. I had to purify and isolate the single factors involved in the process. Lastly, I had to embark on a series of research projects on tumor and cell differentiation biology, and more specifically stem cell biology. This was a huge undertaking, and I needed a research facility that could systematically address these issues.

Because I no longer wished to continue conducting research on animals, I had to set up a new study unit on *in vitro* cultures. I needed professional resources. In those years in Trieste, such resources were lacking after a professor who had started researching *in vitro* tumor cell cultures moved to Turin. The chances for setting up a research group and securing financing were slim, and I soon realized that I would be better off seeking opportunities elsewhere.

While I was weighing my options, I decided to participate in a competition for a post as chief physician of occupational medicine in Milan, and won. I was reluctant to leave Trieste as I had truly fallen in love with the city, its cultural atmosphere, and lifestyle. However, given the challenges I faced in terms of research and the fact that my mother lived near Milan and was growing old, I decided to make the move, much to my mother's joy. I figured maybe there I could find the resources I needed to continue my research. Plus, my mother had been unhappy with my being so far away, and whenever we talked she would beg me to move somewhere closer, so I was happy to fulfill her wish.

With a heavy heart I prepared to leave Trieste and its nostalgic atmosphere. It was a cosmopolitan, open-minded, and sophisticated city, full of cafés where at any given hour you could see women, usually elderly women, alone and placidly enjoying a cigarette or a pipe; where in the silent, sunny afternoons, in the deserted streets of the city center, you could sense Joyce's existential anxiety, Svevo's melancholic irony, the soft whisper of Saba's suffering; and where the friends I had made were selfless, respectful of my freedom, and hoped to see me again sometime in the future.

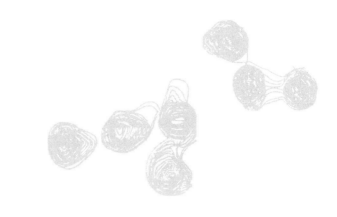

Chapter 5

A Deafening Emptiness

A low, gray, dirty sky so polluted you could see and almost touch it; unbearable noise that gave me constant headaches; chaotic traffic that hindered any movement; an incomprehensible and constant rush of people unaware of their surroundings; no time to prioritize and give meaning to existence; not even the slightest attempt to pause and look at the big picture.

In this deafening emptiness, this crazy race toward nothing, the weight of existence seemed to be more than I could take. Fatigue, strain, and isolation penetrated everything, people's faces and bones. Urban decline permeated every street corner: filth, trash-strewn streets, graffiti scribbles on buildings and monuments, outcasts invisible to the masses, decaying faces of drug addicts, gangs of drug dealers free to roam the city.

And yet the picture of gloom I saw was not one that the city wanted to paint for itself. On the contrary, Milan was depicted as the center of modernity and efficiency, where unparalleled opportunities were available for anyone with the courage to seize them. Frankly, the myth of success and appearances seemed exaggerated to me, and the commercially driven language and mentality of the media worked to contaminate everyone. Even the waiters were on the look-out for a "sponsor," though what sort of sponsorship it was they sought was unclear to me. The contrast between the decay and the image the city wanted to portray hit me like a blow to the gut. One poster that particularly struck me upon my arrival to the city showed the famous Man Ray painting, the one with the smiling red lips suspended in a clear blue sky with billowing clouds, with a phrase at the bottom that read "The future is smiling in Milan."

It was obvious that modernity was unable to recognize its limitations or, if it was, it glossed over them completely by promoting optimism. This circumstance was even more depressing than the despair itself. The weight of this burden drained me of all my energy and quashed any ability to dream. Thank goodness I did not need this place to serve as an inspiration for my discoveries, and luckily my research was based on technical knowledge. This was no place for dreams or imagination, or so I thought. To my surprise, I was mistaken.

After a very difficult break-in period, my relationship with Milan slowly began to improve. I have to say that over time the city itself has improved, or so it seems to me. In fact, now I find it almost beautiful. No doubt it is cleaner and more orderly; the parks and gardens are in better condition and are now suitable places for children to play. There's still the smog and traffic, but this is a problem for all big cities and one that modern society does not seem to know how to confront or solve. There is also still a lot of crime, but there are many people who devote their time and energy to volunteering and helping others which, given the context, makes their effort even more admirable. Milan's problems are those of the modern and post-modern age, and this metropolis is much better than others.

In Milan I had the chance to meet people with lots of energy who have helped me move forward. Organizing the research was time-consuming—not everything was smooth sailing and unfortunately many years were wasted. However, in the end, we have been able to establish a facility with gifted people with whom in just a few years a great deal of work has been completed. Many aspects of the problems that I intended to tackle have been clarified, so that now the overall picture is fairly clear. Thanks to the scientific articles that we have published, we are now known by other research groups and can establish steady collaborations that are ongoing, such as the one with the La Sapienza University in Rome, where three departments are currently working on this branch of research.

The Outcome of Research

As planned from the start, all our research was conducted on *in vitro* cancer cell cultures. Eight different types of human tumors were used: multiform glioblastoma (a brain tumor), breast tumor, liver tumor, kidney tumor, colon tumor, uterine tumor, melanoma, and acute lymphoblastic leukemia.

To assess the effects on tumor growth of the administration of cellular differentiation factors, we first had to choose which embryo to use as a study model for differentiation and development. The three embryos most often studied are *Drosophila melanogaster* (which we had already used in previous experiments), *Xenophus laevis* (frog), and *Brachydanio rerio* (more commonly known as the zebrafish, a small, striped tropical fish). Today *Caenorhabditis elegans*, a tiny nematode roundworm, is also widely studied. Having to evaluate the effects of factors extracted from embryos of ovoviviparous animals on human tumors, we had to choose embryos that from a phylogenetic (i.e., evolutionary) viewpoint are most similar to man.

We immediately ruled out the Drosophila (which we had already used in our previous experiments on mice, but only for contingent reasons), because it is phylogenetically distant from humans. In a choice between zebrafish and Xenophus, having learned in our labs that they had common antigens and cellular receptors maintained during phylogenesis, in the end we chose to use the zebrafish, for a variety of reasons.

First, they are easy to raise. The water temperature in their aquariums must be kept within a precise range, but in fact this is very simple to do. Second, it is easy to precisely establish the moment of fertilization. For our experiment this element was vitally important, as we needed to understand when the cells differentiated and when they merely multiplied. Later I will clarify why knowing the precise moment of fertilization is so important. In any event, fertilization of zebrafish eggs occurs at dawn. Therefore, by planning dark/light cycles it is easy to determine when fertilization will take place. Furthermore, as a result of the studies conducted on zebrafish, all the images of the embryo within the different brief intervals of development have been published. By comparing the microscopic images of an embryo extracted at a given moment and the images published, it is easy to determine and double-check exactly when fertilization occurred.

Moreover, studies on zebrafish embryos have made it possible to identify somewhat precisely when important differentiation is occurring. In that moment several genes switch on and off, a sign that the genoma is undergoing substantial changes in gene expression. Previous studies on zebrafish embryos have allowed us to identify and choose three moments in which important cell differentiation takes place: the moments of embryonic development chosen correspond to the start of cellular differentiation, for example, the brief period in which totipotent embryonic stem cells differentiate and become pluripotent. (Later as the characteristics of the terms I use become clearer, so will the stem-cell terminology.) Two other moments of differentiation chosen include one in the intermediate phase and the other in the final phase of embryonic development.

Finally, we also wanted to study what happens to human tumors when factors are administrated that have been extracted from embryos when they multiply without differentiating. Therefore we also selected a phase of embryonic development in which only multiplication occurs. We chose embryos before they started to differentiate and, more specifically, when they were composed only of totipotent embryonic stem cells. The experiments were conducted and repeated many times in order to ensure reliable results.

It emerged that certain factors present at the time of stem-cell differentiation are able to slow down or inhibit tumor growth. However, these factors are present only at the moment in which the stem cells differentiate and not when they multiply. The material collected from the zebrafish embryo when it is made up solely of totipotent embryonic stem cells that have not yet differentiated not only does not slow down the multiplication of tumor cells, it encourages their proliferation. This is why, as I already mentioned, it so important to know exactly when fertilization occurs.

This finding is in line with literature data on the risks of the occurrence of cancerous diseases when totipotent embryonic stem cells are used in experiments to treat certain pathologies. Therefore, it follows that tumor growth is arrested during differentiation. Molecular mechanisms responsible for slowing tumor growth differ depending on the type of tumor, but all share a single, fundamental element: they all stop the cellular cycle. This occurs because fundamental molecules that control the cellular cycle mechanism, such as the p53 tumor suppressor gene and retinoblastoma protein (pRb), are regulated by stem-cell differentiation factors. As a result, cancer multiplication is arrested, and as this occurs genetic damage at the origin of the disease is repaired and the cells differentiate or, if the mutations cannot be repaired, genes prompting programmed cell death (apoptosis) are activated and the cells die. Lab studies have shown that cancer cell apoptosis and re-differentiation increase when differentiation factors are added to tumor cells, as is evidenced in the sharp rise of differentiation markers such as E-caderin. In practice, differentiation factors have the same function and role in regard to cancer cells as embryos.

Various studies have demonstrated that the p53 tumor suppressor gene is activated every time the embryo genoma undergoes a mutation or cancerous insult. Essentially, this is the corrective system I had visualized in Trieste that evening on the pier in the yellow-orange light. This gene has even been called the "guardian of babies" because it nips embryonic mutation in the bud and prevents it from becoming dangerous and causing tumors in children.

However, when the genetic insult to the embryo is massive, the p53 tumor suppressor gene is no longer able to repair DNA damage.

As a result, instead of allowing the cancer to arise, it causes apoptosis, i.e., programmed cell death (miscarriage). This is also what happens with cancer cells when they are put into contact with stem-cell differentiation factors. Either the damage is repaired and the cells re-differentiate, or the damage is so serious that it cannot be repaired and the cells die.

Our research therefore showed that cancer cells are "educated" to behave in a physiological manner. Instead of being destroyed in a war that would be too risky and dangerous, they are educated to differentiate, like all the tissues of the human body, or die spontaneously.

From this standpoint cancer is a reversible pathology. These experiments made it possible for us to prepare a product for all intents and purposes in its infancy. The product contains low doses of differentiation factors and has been clinically tested. This product was prepared in the form of a solution to be taken orally. Since the active fraction that arrests tumor development has a very low molecular weight, sub-lingual administration seemed to be the most appropriate. A controlled, randomized clinical study was conducted from 1 January 2001 to 31 April 2004 on 179 patients with an intermediate or advanced phase of primitive liver cancer against which no other therapy was possible. (The use of the product was therefore compassionate. At our current state of clinical studies, this product must still be used in advanced cancer diseases.) The results were published in *Oncology Research* in December 2005.

More recently, our research was confirmed in the summer of 2006, when a publication appeared in *Nature Medicine* that pleased me very much. Some colleagues at the Children's Hospital of Chicago implanted a highly malignant and aggressive melanoma in a zebrafish embryo, the same tropical fish that I had been using in our labs for the last fifteen years. The same melanoma was also implanted in adult fish. The tumors implanted in the embryos did not develop, but because they gave rise to different tissue, they enabled the formation of normal fish, while the tumors implanted in the adult organisms developed significantly. The researchers concluded that the embryonic microenvironment was able to control tumor growth and inhibit it through regulatory processes.

When the researchers at the Children's Hospital of Chicago found out about our lab experiments they congratulated us. Professor Mary J.C. Hendrix, the President of the Children's Hospital, invited us to Chicago. Obviously we were very happy about the invitation, but mostly about the fact that zebrafish embryos had "saved" themselves and were living examples that confirmed our many experiments.

While on the one side the role of stem-cell differentiation factors in the control of tumor growth has been confirmed, on the other side further research on factors produced by the uterus during pregnancy has led to the isolation of a low-weight molecular fraction, the so-called "Life-Protecting Factor" that is able to counteract tumor growth by provoking programmed cell death. This fraction is produced by the mother at a very early stage. We isolated it in the moment in which in the embryo's totipotent stem cells are undergoing differentiation. There is an ongoing cross-talk between the mother and the embryo at a very early stage, before the various organs and systems, including the brain, begin to differentiate. Even before the embryo is formed the mother identifies the stem cells that are creating life, a being different from herself.

This fact is significant in terms of ethics and is an issue I will address further on in the text. For now, suffice to say that sometimes life hides many surprises, and reality is much more intricate and complex than we suspect. For this reason, I think one should be careful in saying that an embryo can be considered a new life only when the brain has formed. What is thought to be a group of stem cells is in fact something very different: it is a newly emerging life. It is a new being and the mother knows this, not in the metaphoric but in the literal sense of the term. These concepts will become clearer when I deal with the issue of communication in biology.

In conclusion, at the origin of life a myriad of events take place that in some way are able to fight cancer. Why stem-cell differentiation factors are able to arrest the multiplication of cancer cells and what diseases fall under the name of cancer are questions I will answer in the following chapters.

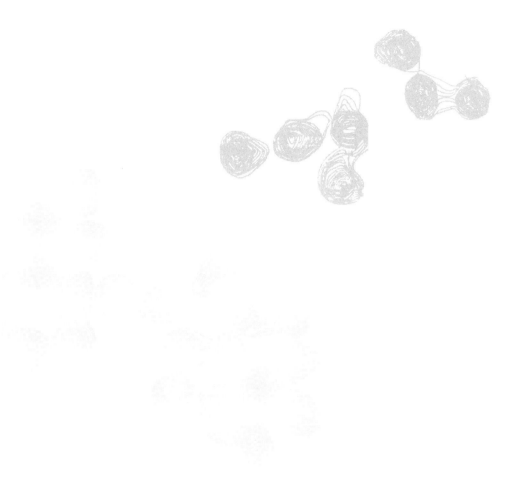

Chapter 6

Calculations in Duomo Square

One pleasant Sunday morning in April—perhaps one of the best months in Milan, as it's not too cold and not too hot and soft breezes clear the air—my wife and I decided to take a walk to the Duomo Cathedral. We wanted to browse the bookshops in the Vittorio Emanuele Gallery.

I had just finished reading a publication on embryonic differentiation by Stuart Kauffman, a biologist and evolutionist at the Santa Fe Institute. Kauffman had been very courageous in proposing a model on the crucial process through which life is created. Given the enormously complex factors involved, the mere thought of the possibility of embarking on such a vast undertaking is mind-boggling. And yet Kauffman had succeeded in presenting a most interesting model that interpreted reality coherently.

His model is made up of binary networks (Booleans) composed of a certain number (N) of nodes (capable of switching "on" and "off") and a certain number of inputs (K) for each node. Kauffman demonstrated with this model that, given certain rules of commutation, in the case of K>2 the network of embryonic genes is in a chaotic state, but if K is nearer to 2, the network becomes stable and organizes itself in a dynamic order. Around frozen nodes—ones that as the system goes through a cycle remain in the same state of activation or configuration—non-frozen "islands" are formed in which the behavior of the network is not crystallized (static order) or sensitive to the butterfly effect, which I mentioned earlier, as occurs in chaotic systems.

What was also very interesting in Kauffman's publication was the observation that the network of embryonic genes not only is stable and orderly, it is the result of a process involving relatively few cycles. In addition, the number of genetic configurations, in other words of differentiated cells, is also relatively low (slightly above 300), indeed not so far from 252, which is the number of cell types that effectively compose all the organs and systems of the human body. Basically, Kauffman's model of embryonic differentiation shows that life is created through processes characterized by converging trajectories, and that at the limit of chaos a gratuitous order emerges.

The article had piqued my interest, and as I walked with my wife that morning I told her about it. I wanted her take on it, and since she has a degree in mathematics she could explain some of the more complex notions that I hadn't completely understood and could help me better evaluate the reach of the publication. My wife has the uncanny ability to make me understand logic and mathematics; if I had had her as a teacher when I was younger, I probably would have liked math much more.

I told her how the number of cell types had been calculated and we focused our attention on 252, the number of cell types actually counted within the human body. I suggested that we try to calculate the number not on the basis of a purely theoretical model, but based on new knowledge acquired on embryo differentiation.

To do this the entire process of embryonic development had to be examined by starting *ad ovo* or rather from the fertilized egg (the cell) that is created from the union of two sex cells, one male and one female, and that therefore contains the genetic material (hereditary information) of both parents.*

Embryo Development

Let's start by examining the stages of development, which, in the creation of a multi-cellular being, begin at the time the egg is fer-

---

Note: This chapter has been simplified for a wide readership. A more detailed, although still summarized, explanation of the biological events responsible for embryo development and differentiation can be found in the Appendix at the end of this book.

tilized. Development involves processes of cellular multiplication and differentiation, i.e., specialization.

The human body is made up of about one quadrillion cells, most of which carry out highly specialized functions that derive from a single cell, the fertilized egg. All these processes occur in the embryo at a rate that requires a surprising amount of coherency. All cells are linked in a precise and flexible manner to each other. Without a level of coherency equivalent to that found in embryos, the organization of life would not be possible. The processes of cell replication and specialization occur through a series of complex stages (which I summarize below) that take place at mind-boggling speed.

In the first stage, the embryo develops from a single cell: the fertilized egg. The processes of development on the one side include multiplicative events that enable the embryo to grow and acquire a certain body mass, and on the other differentiation events that enable the cells to specialize and form tissue and organs (kidney, liver, brain, lung, etc.). The processes of differentiation that lead to undifferentiated totipotent cells, in which completely undifferentiated cells multiply rapidly, are highly selective processes through which specialization is directly related to the progressive inability to multiply. The differentiation processes allow the genes to be regulated specifically and selectively (genes intended as a macromolecule of deoxyribonucleic acid—DNA—able to induce the synthesis of specific proteins), thereby determining which ones should remain active and which ones should not. The genes remaining active at the end of the process are responsible for the synthesis of specific proteins on the basis of which specific tissues that make up various organs are characterized. The difference among the various tissue cells is determined by which specific genes have remained active and therefore by which specific proteins are synthesized. Consequently, at the end of differentiation, all the differentiated cells will have the same initial DNA (that of the fertilized egg) but the fraction of active genome responsible for codifying the proteins will be different in each specialized cell. The regulation processes of genes that codify proteins are activated by a tight network of molecules that together make up an "epigenetic code." This code enables a totipotent embryonic stem cell (the origin of all cells) to become a liver cell, kidney cell, brain cell, lung cell, etc., thereby determining which codifying gene should remain active and which should not.

Besides containing the genes responsible for codifying proteins, the genome also contains large portions of DNA that until a few years ago were referred to as "junk DNA." We have learned, however, that junk DNA in fact plays an important role in regulating codifying DNA. This fact emerged thanks to the sequencing of the genetic code. As a result, we discovered that for example in the human species less than two percent of the genetic code, totaling roughly 21,000 genes, is needed to codify proteins. Before the start of the sequencing process, it was estimated that there were between 80,000 and 100,000 codifying human genes. The relatively low number of 21,000 genes (in fact only slightly higher than that of the fruit fly) goes to show that the diversity observed in the protein molecules (which in humans number approximately 100,000) is the result of differing regulation processes of single genes. In superior organisms, such as humans, greater complexity is associated with a higher regulation capacity, rather than a higher quantity of codifying genes. A medium-sized gene in reality codifies more than a protein molecule. Indeed, the genes of certain organisms can codify more than 3,000 different proteins.

In a cell, in addition to the codifying genetic code, there is also a tight-knit network of molecules and a substantial portion of DNA that perform regulatory functions. This is in fact also a code, known as the "epigenetic code" (mentioned above). This code makes up the precise system that regulates gene expression during embryonic development and therefore makes it possible for the cell to differentiate and specialize. Just as the conductor of an orchestra decides how a piece of music is to be played, so the epigenetic code determines how the codifying DNA within each cell should be read. With the exception of very few cases, the differences between specialized cells are epigenetic and not genetic. Today the study of epigenetics is changing the face of biology. The twenty-first century launches the era of epigenetics, shifting the spotlight that was previously focused solely on the genetic code.

We still do not realize the extent of these changes and their implications for further research, even if the prospects for the future in the therapeutic field are likely to stem from this branch of research rather than from genetics, where results linked to genetic manipulation have been disappointing and ethically questionable. Especially after the discovery of microRNA (ribonucleic acid) with regulatory functions, a new world emerged filled with highly promising therapeutic prospects.

MicroRNA are small molecules of ribonucleic acid made up of 21 to 23 nucleotides (the building blocks of RNA) that are able to regulate codifying genes through complex mechanisms (see Appendix for further details). MiRNA is involved in cell differentiation and has a significant impact on the regulation of gene expression and therefore on the development of an organism.

Studies in which a part of the machinery of miRNA processing was destroyed have shown that an organism cannot survive without the regulator role that miRNA plays. Through interfering with RNA it is possible to virtually deactivate in a selective manner any gene simply by introducing a miRNA inside a cell. The potential benefits arising from the application of this technique are enormous.

As I mentioned earlier, through the regulatory mechanisms of gene expression, the embryo develops and differentiates. In actual fact, during the first stages of development the embryo multiplies without differentiating. The fertilized egg multiplies through a process of "symmetrical" cellular division in which each mother cell divides into two daughter cells that are identical to the mother.

This leads to the formation of the structure called a morula (berry) because of its shape. The two daughter cells are called totipotent embryonic stem cells because they can give rise to any kind of cell and therefore give life to a new being.

After this multiplicative phase the cells begin to differentiate and a blastocyst is formed—a structure made up of an internal mass of cells that develops into an embryo from a hollow cavity surrounded by a layer of cells. In mammals this cell layer becomes the embryonic membrane and placenta.

In this stage not all embryonic cells are totipotent, because the ones surrounding the blastocyst that develop embryonic membranes now start to differentiate. The totipotent cells of the internal mass of the blastocyst also start to differentiate into daughter cells, which give rise to three primary germ cell layers: ectoderm (which will develop into the skin, including mammary tissue and the nervous system), endoderm (which will develop into the tissue of the digestive system, including the digestive glands), and mesoderm (which will develop into bones, muscle, connective tissue, and blood vessels). The cell's loss of totipotency and gain of specialized functions is the consequence of an asymmetric division (the mother cells on the one hand spawn identical daughter cells and on the other differing cells that have begun to differentiate). Subsequent divisions will create different types of stem cells which, according to their degree of specialization, will be defined as: a) pluripotent; b) multipotent; c) oligopotent; d) definitively differentiating cells; or e) completely differentiated cells. It should be pointed out that these cells gradually acquire specialized functions and progressively lose their ability to multiply. Indeed, completely differentiated cells are no longer able to multiply. Cells that in certain tissue of adult organisms continue to multiply and then differentiate—such as bone marrow cells, cells that develop into blood cells, skin germ cells, or intestinal villus cells—are in fact stem cells that remain in an adult organism.

How many cell differentiation stages does a human embryo undergo? To answer this question we must return to the initial problem: to the question that my wife and I had asked ourselves during our walk to the Cathedral that Sunday morning in April.

Based on the conclusions we have reached so far, we can say that a cell undergoes five differentiation stages: the totipotent stage, pluripotent stage, oligopotent stage, etc., until the cell has differentiated completely. Obviously five is an average figure as the number could be higher or lower depending on the type of cell. Five is a reasonable number that could roughly indicate reality.

Now, if we consider what happens in the embryo at the initial stage of differentiation when ectoderm, endoderm, and mesoderm (the three primary germ cell layers) are formed—in other words when a common parent with three different regulation programs for gene expression gives rise to three daughter cells in three types of asymmetric, obviously different, divisions—and if we assume that this model is the basis for subsequent stages of cell differentiation, then the number of various cell types that make up the human body can be achieved through a simple mathematical formula:

$$3^5$$

Three (the number of events that occur in each stage of differentiation) to the power of five (the number of times in which the event repeats itself). The result is 243 somatic cells. If to this number we add the number of cell types that derive from the germinative line (nine: four females—oogonium, primary oocyte, secondary oocyte, and the differentiated egg cell—and five males—spermatogonium, primary spermatocytes, secondary spermatocytes, spermatids, and spermatozoa), which differentiate themselves differently from other somatic cells, the number of different cell types of the human species is 252, which is the exact number counted. The three cell daughters arising from the common parent cell is also meant to be understood as an average number, since for some types of cells this number could be higher while for other types, especially toward the end of embryonic differentiation, lower. (In the final stages of cell differentiation the cells that have progressively lost their mul-tipotency in some cases become unipotent. So you see how three—the number of daughter cells arising from a common parent cell—is merely an average number.)

What is fascinating is that life, so complex in its vastness, is based on such a simple algorithm. This surprised my wife and me as we made our way toward Piazza Cordusio and identified the mathe-matical formula to summarize what occurs in the embryo during cell differentiation. This was cause for celebration so before we reached the bookshop in Vittorio Emanuele Gallery we stopped for a drink at Camparino.

Chapter 7

Closer to Solving the Enigma

The following Monday morning I thought I would verify whether the idea I had come up with the day before with my wife could be used to calculate the number of different types of human tumors. The tumors that fall under the name of cancer are in fact different diseases that share certain pathogenetic mechanisms. The thought that the embryonic differentiation process could take place in a limited number of stages had got me to thinking that maybe it was possible to build a cancer model that could explain what cancer is.

In essence, the idea had sparked within me the thought that I could create a model that could explain and reclassify the various types of tumors and shed light on many mysteries surrounding these diseases. After all the experiments I had conducted and all the thought given and studies performed on stem-cell differentiation, it was becoming increasingly clear to me what these diseases referred to as "cancer" actually were. I felt that I had acquired the information I needed to put together the pieces of the puzzle to compose a picture in which all tumor diseases could find a place and an explanation. Thus, I set out to link the pieces. Many things were already widely known.

The Causes of Cancer

For some time now we have known that the causes of more than ninety percent of tumors are related to the environment, and the remaining ten percent are due to disease arising from viruses or inherited pathologies, such as retinoblastoma, a rare tumor. We also know that tumors inherited at birth are rare, whereas cases in which heredity causes a greater predisposition to cancer are more frequent.

Among the leading causes of cancer is lifestyle—for example, smoking or diet. We know that a high-calorie diet high in fat and red meat and low in fiber increases the risk of cancer. A low-calorie diet low in fat and red meat and high in fruit, vegetables, and fiber and high-protein foods such as seeds and beans and certain types of algae or fish can protect against cancer.

Cancer-causing environmental factors include air, water, and soil pollution that indirectly contaminate the food we eat. In large cities researchers have found roughly 3,000 chemical pollutants, of which around 50 have been classified as certain, probable, or possible cancer-causing agents. The certain carcinogens include physical agents such as ionizing radiation, while suspected agents include electromagnetic radiation. Exposure to environmental carcinogens is often work-related. For example, pleuric mesothelioma, which I studied in my research on environmentally related cancers in Trieste, is mainly a work-related pathology arising from exposure to asbestos, which fortunately has been eliminated from production cycles. Stress and depression are other contributing factors to cancer.

Many agencies around the world study and classify the various causes of cancer. Among these perhaps the most famous is the IARC (International Agency for Research on Cancer), a World Health Organization agency based in Lyon, France. The IARC publishes a series of monographs that gathers literature data from around the world and subjects papers to a systematic critical review. The monograph program of the IARC started in 1971 and analyzes each carcinogenic or suspected carcinogenic substance in three phases: a) collecting all the data possible to evaluate the cancer risk; b) critically analyzing the data with the help of expert international committees; and c) publishing and divulging the results in the form of monographs. For a chemical substance to be analyzed the agency determines whether or not the agent is proven or suspected to cause cancer in humans or is proven to cause cancer in animals exposed to the agent. Just because a substance has not been analyzed in an

IARC monograph does not mean that it is free of cancer risk. Until now the IARC has examined only a fraction of existing chemical substances and industrial processes. Millions of known chemical substances and several thousand agents manufactured and sold each year have not been analyzed. Keeping this in mind, for the sake of completeness, I have included after the Appendix a table listing the certain carcinogens for humans as identified to date by the IARC.

Another key issue in the discussion on carcinogens is the experimentally clear evidence that has led researchers to conclude that merely the smallest dose of carcinogen, even if completely metabolized and eliminated by the organism, has irreversible effects that summed together will clinically manifest as cancer. Doses, including small ones, sometimes require a long latency period from the first exposure to the clinical manifestation of a tumor. For this reason neoplastic diseases appear late in life, as they are infantile tumors that are usually due to the fetus' (not embryo's) exposure to an environmental carcinogen.

The question remains: how do carcinogens give rise to tumors?

The Mechanism Responsible for Cancer Genesis

The initial mechanism of the process is often a mutation that may slightly or severely alter DNA. Fortunately a mutation is not sufficient to cause disease, otherwise tumors would be much more widespread than they already are today.

It is believed that the transformation of a normal cell into a cancer cell is a process involving chance mutational events ranging between four and seven in number. If the mutations are induced in the cell on a non-chance basis—for example, if specific genes are targeted—this number could be reduced. These mutations seem to specifically target genes that codify proteins with a key role in regulating the cellular cycle and in cellular signaling, as well as microRNA regulators and growth factors with their receptors.

Defining the transformation of a normal cell into a cancer cell simply as the result of a sum of mutations could be reductive. The transformation relies on a complex network of signals between cells that "speak to each other" or on soluble extracellular factors. As a case in point, it has been proven that certain cells (such as fibroblasts) that are adjacent to tumor cells (such as epithelial carcinoma) are able to direct tumor progression. Furthermore, evidence has shown that cells near connective structures are able to promote the transformation of immortalized cells by releasing a proliferating stimulus, and that cells connected by inflammatory processes can withstand, instead of fight, tumor growth. This overall context is fundamental in determining the fate of a cell in line with a wide scope of cellular biology. In keeping with this outlook, cancer genesis could be rightly defined as a microevolutive process. As a consequence of this process tumor cells acquire the ability to: a) be self-sufficient in growth signals; b) be insensitive to signals that block growth; c) survive and avoid apoptosis (programmed cellular death); d) potentially replicate without limit; e) maintain the continued formation of new blood vessels (angiogenesis); and f) invade tissues and give rise to metastasis. These abilities are usually the result of an enormous variability in mechanisms that, as in the initial phase of transformation, cells use to become malignant. There is no precise or clear-cut process through which normal cells become cancer. Many different types of mutations and many different types of contexts can lead to cancer.

The experiments conducted in our lab, however, demonstrated that despite the large variations among these genetic processes and contexts, the development of all types of human tumors is governed by a common final process. Some authors refer to the transformations that make a cell accumulate genetic mutations as "early crisis." Some of these crises can be overcome given the fact that at cellular level there are mechanisms that control genetic damage, such as the checkpoint p53. As I have already mentioned, in the event of a mutation, the p53 protein blocks the cellular cycle and induces the transcription of a p21 protein, which repairs damaged DNA. If the mutations are non-repairable, genes are activated to induce apoptosis. As a result of this checkpoint, the cell may either die or survive. If it survives, it can still undergo other mutations and then initiate a process of chaotic bifurcation. These are the paths the cell can take based on slight changes in context. Small variations are enough to change the final result of the checkpoints. Once triggered, the chaotic process can continue a series of multiple bifurcations that, if the cell does not die, can give rise to rampant genetic instability. At this point, the cell would continue in its path until a point that some researchers call "genetic catastrophe," when the cell becomes a tumor cell and, according to widely held scientific opinion, pursues a path of uncontrollable chaos with no purpose. As this path is absolutely out of control and has no objective, the only way to stop it is to provoke the suppression of the cells that become tumor cells.

Today all research is based on this assumption and geared toward identifying molecules and other means to inhibit the tumor by destroying it more or less selectively. Recent important steps in this direction have been made leading to therapies that are more specific and selective than traditional chemotherapy, which uses multiclonal antibodies, angiogenesis inhibitors, or enzyme inhibitors that trigger the cellular cycle, as well as proteasome inhibitors so the cells accumulate rejection proteins that cause the tumor's death.

The research carried out in our labs has shown that a chaotic process that later stabilizes leads to cancer. The process is stabilized by what the chaos theory refers to as an "attractor" that leads the genome of the tumor cell to a new configuration. Depending on the degree of malignancy, the configuration is similar to that present in the embryo in different stages of development. If the cell were not to stabilize it would not even be possible to classify different types of tumors. Our experiments have shown that tumor cells are mutated stem cells. The factors that differentiate stem cells are capable of differentiating or causing apoptosis even in tumor cells by bypassing the mutations that are at the source of the malignancy.

Tumor cells and stem cells share many similarities. First of all, they both have active embryonic genes that are responsible for cellular multiplication. These are called proto-oncogenes. These genes are "turned off" during the differentiation process and for this reason are not active in completely differentiated cells. In tumor cells, these genes are often mutated and thus are called oncogenes. They are responsible for multiplication events as they produce embryonic growth factors. In addition, in tumor cells the genes responsible for the arrest of multiplication are often mutated and deactivated. These genes are known as oncosuppressor genes, one example being the p53 gene, as I have already mentioned. In this case, there is no brake in tumor growth. On the one side, tumor cells deactivate growth stop signals, and on the other side they activate growth factors. It should be pointed out that several tumor growth factors, including those responsible for the formation of blood vessels (angiogenesis), are in actual fact embryonic growth factors. Moreover, tumor cells have several membrane antigens known as oncofetal antigens, so called because they are present also in embryo cells. These antigens are the likely receptors to which differentiation factors hook onto and send growth stop signals within the cell. Finally, unlike other cells, they both have an anaerobic metabolism that does not entail the use of oxygen. I should also clarify that as soon as a cell has activated certain oncogenes and deactivated certain oncosuppressors, it undergoes uncontrollable multiplication, not unlike a car traveling at maximum speed with no brakes.

Other similarities between tumor and embryo cells are their metabolic paths and molecular effectors. Some paths have very strange names like the APC/beta catenina/TCF/WNT path and the Hedgehog/Smoothened/Patched path shared by both types of cells.

In embryo development these paths lead to successful cell differentiation. In tumor cells the mutated counterparts lead the cell to continuous and indefinite multiplication. This occurs because the tumor cell is undifferentiated such that the mutations present in its genome do not enable it to complete the entire differentiation and development process. This is blocked in a phase of the multiplication process, in between two stages of differentiation. The tumor cell can therefore be defined as a "mutated stem cell" in which on one side there is an imbalance of the epigenetic code in an embryonic sense, and on the other side mutations occur that have split the differentiation and multiplication programs. It is important to understand these two aspects and the fact that in cancer alterations to the genetic code and epigenetic code occur.

Currently researchers' attention is focused on the genetic alterations of cancer. It is important to map as much as possible the various genetic alterations, but this is not enough. This is a limited and short-sighted vision of cancer. Mutations are not enough to give rise to cancer. It is the imbalance of the epigenetic code in the embryonic sense, together with the various alterations of this code, that make tumor cells take on the characteristics of an embryonic cell. These conclusions are not based on purely theoretical speculation but are supported by experiments conducted in our labs on the stem-cell differentiation factors. Our experiments have shown among other things that the cancer model (see Figure 1) is not a theoretical hypothesis but an experimentally verified model.

Having explored the paths aimed at regulating gene expression in tumor cells, we can now summarize the knowledge we have gathered and propose the model shown in Figure 1.

Unless these concepts are taken into account in their entirety, it will be difficult to find a therapeutic strategy that breaks free from the traditional therapeutic mindset centered on destroying tumor cells, with all the negative side-effects that this entails. The use of stem-cell differentiation factors is based on a very strong rationale.

Legend

A: normal cell **B**: cell with damaged DNA **C**: cell with rampant genetic instability
D: cancer cell: stable gene configuration with uncoupled steps of cell multiplication and differentiation
E: multipotent stem cell **F**: oligopotent stem cell **G**: differentiating cell **H**: differentiated cell

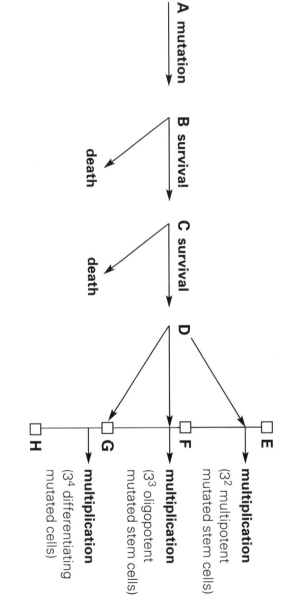

Figure 1: CANCER AS A PROCESS OF DETERMINISTIC CHAOS

We aim to correct the imbalance of the epigenetic code and re-establish the cell's ability to differentiate, bypassing the mutations that are at the origin of the malignancy.

Our differentiation therapy does not seek to destroy the cells in a war-like fashion, at the expense of the individual's health and safety, but instead wishes to "teach and educate" the cells to return to their normal physiology and organismic context. If we compare this to information technology, we can say that this therapy re-sets within the tumor cells the codifying DNA's altered hard disk and installs a new program of cell differentiation, i.e., a correct epigenetic program.

So much attention today is focused on the role of microRNAs in relation to embryo development and cancer. We are starting to understand that it is possible to silence specific messengerRNAs using specific microRNAs, making it possible to indirectly modify the gene expression of various forms of cancer. However, single or just a few microRNAs will unfortunately not be sufficient for this purpose. We will need more or less complex cocktails given the seriousness of the imbalance of the microRNA network in cancer and the sheer amount of alterations that need to be corrected. Therefore, using the factors present during stem-cell differentiation (which at that stage contain regulating proteins of the gene expression and microRNAs) is, paradoxically and taken as a whole, a simplification of the challenges facing cancer treatment. Just as it is easier to achieve beneficial results for the body by consuming all the factors and vitamins contained, say, in fruit, rather than ingesting single vitamins or single factors, likewise it is probably much easier to gain positive results by using a pool of epigenetic regulation factors extracted during the various phases of cell differentiation. Nature itself teaches us what to do; all we have to do is observe it and understand.

At this point, the challenge in cancer treatment will be to identify exactly which pool of regulation factors should be used for a given tumor. To do this, we must find out how many types of tumors exist, as each type will likely require its own epigenetic regulation network.

Types of Tumors

An embryo differentiation model can be useful to help us understand how many types of tumors exist. If the tumor cells are undifferentiated mutated cells, the number can be calculated keeping in mind the differentiation model my wife and I devised during our walk on that Sunday in April.

According to this model, tumor cells are obviously represented by all types of cells undergoing differentiation and present in the embryo until the final differentiation phase, before complete cell differentiation. In this case, the mathematical formula for calculating the number of types of tumors deriving from cells that give rise to all body tissue, with the exception of sex cells, is as follows:

$$N = 3+3^2+3^3+3^4 = 120$$

To calculate the final number of tumor types, it is necessary to add to 120 the number of tumors that derive from germ cells (which give rise to sex cells and differentiate in a different manner than somatic cells) and from different embryonic tissue (teratocarcinoma, corioncarcinoma, embryonic carcinoma). The final sum of all types of tumors therefore is approximately 130. Figure 1, already presented, shows the stages of the deterministic chaos leading up to the final attractor that transforms normal cells into different kinds of cancer.

In terms of malignancy, the most aggressive tumors are those with genetic configurations present in the first stages of embryonic differentiation in which the cell multiplies at mind-boggling speed. For example, very aggressive leukemias, such as lymphoblastic and myeloid leukemias, are composed of mutated multi-potent stem cells that multiply much faster than differentiating cells present in chronic lymphatic leukemia.

The current classifications of tumors are redundant because they do not consider that from an ontogenetic viewpoint, as a tumor that originates in a specific organ becomes increasingly aggressive it flows into cell types that share the same genetic configuration with tumors in other organs. Finally, we must bear in mind that some tumor types are made up of differing cellular clones with varying degrees of malignancy and thus of cells with genetic configurations that derive from various stages of differentiation.

As you can see, the model adequately explains what exactly cancer is. Cancer is made up of around 130 different diseases (maybe more, as 130 is the number calculated according to a model, which, as such, is a simplification of reality) in which cells have been altered, due to the mutation of the genetic code and to an imbalance of the epigenetic code, and transformed into mutated stem cells.

What visibly emerges is the fact that the cancer model I am presenting clearly shows all the various cell types that are at the basis of the various cancers. In this model, the tumors cease to be mysterious diseases whose fundamental alterations are not understood, and everything is sufficiently explained. From an ontogenetic standpoint, the processes that lead to cancer are clarified, thereby enabling the conception of new therapeutic approaches, especially in the field of so-called differentiation therapies, geared toward "educating" tumor cells to evolve toward normal development. Each tumor type could be treated this way with its own specific therapy.

The road we have embarked on in our labs could be further pursued to perfect the therapies that we are currently implementing and that have given noteworthy results (which, as already mentioned, are described in a forty-month-long randomized controlled clinical study in 179 patients affected with advanced-stage primitive liver cancer, and published in *Oncology Research* in 2005).

The therapies we have conceived and begun to implement can be improved by identifying precisely which fractions of differentiation factors are more specifically active on different tumor types. In this way, we could lay the foundation for individualized cancer therapy. From the pool of differentiation factors we could arrive at specific therapies. The road is complex, but it would simplify problems.

Another road similar to the one we have undertaken, but which would be undoubtedly longer and more complicated (not complex), is the one that is starting to emerge after the discovery of microRNA. We can map the genetic and epigenetic alterations that cause cancer and then attempt regulation and modulation therapies to re-establish balance within the severely imbalanced microRNA network. This is a complicated process from various viewpoints. First, it would be necessary to identify at least the main genes involved in the mutations of each specific tumor type. Second, what type of imbalance is present in the microRNA network or what alterations exist in the composition of the network would have to be verified. Third, keeping in mind that often tumors affecting an individual are made up of differing cell clones, it would be necessary to establish which aforementioned alterations are specific to each individual clone. Last but not least, during therapy cells often adapt to treatment by finding a way of becoming resistant to it; in this case we would be back to square one.

This approach to cancer might very well be pursued in the future, but it will be a long time before it can be applied. Now, however, we can begin studying how to apply this approach to tumorous disease, where the imbalance of the microRNA network is not too severely altered. For instance, in chronic lymphatic leukemia we are starting to see a road open up in this direction.

The road my group has taken has led to interesting initial clinical results and is one that can be pursued in a relatively short time. Of course, our approach to cancer can and must be perfected. As already noted, our approach envisages the use of factors present in the initial, intermediate, and final stages of stem-cell differentiation.

These differentiation factors are capable of deactivating genes that have been reactivated during the cancer genesis process and that have made tumor cells similar to mutated stem cells.

In other words, ours is an epigenetic tumor therapy that aims to repair cell damage and reprogram cells so that they can undergo normal development. This is why differentiation factors work in regulating processes that lead to normalization or apoptosis of tumor cells. Nature has seen to fully composing the puzzle of these factors, so why undo it and then risk putting it back together incompletely or wrongly? In terms of research, I see no problem in taking an analytical approach—as any specific knowledge is always useful—but if there is a shorter way, then why not pursue it right now? Of course, sizable investments would be needed to make the treatments more effective, but it would very well be worth it.

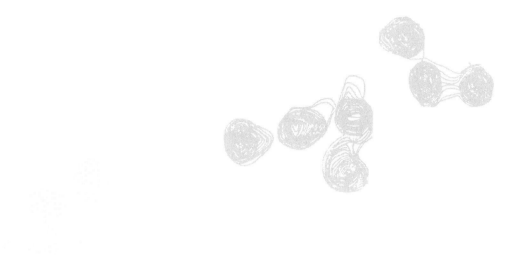

Chapter 8

The Complex Reality of Life

Rudolf Steiner, the founder of anthroposophy, beautifully defines the cognitive process in his book *The Philosophy of Freedom*. For Steiner, knowledge is the process through which the self unites with the universe. In this process rationality, willingness, and sensibility (self-awareness) act in unison to obtain the type of knowledge Steiner refers to. Rationality is not the only factor in the process of knowledge. When unbound by willingness and sensibility, rationality leads to a kind of knowledge that does not connect you with the world but instead creates barriers between the self and the world: to objectify knowledge is to create a dividing wall between us and reality so that we lose our sense of belonging to the world. We become unaware of our link with the world and see ourselves as being outside and not inside the universe.

Achieving the knowledge that Steiner speaks of is a difficult task, especially in the field of exact sciences, to which biology should strive to belong. In actual fact, quantum physics has taught us that in the process of knowledge it is impossible to separate the object of knowledge from the subject that initiates the cognitive process, and Heisenberg's principle of indetermination should become a common heritage of all fields of knowledge. Besides this principle, other extremely problematic moments of cognitive processes have been identified. Given that acquiring knowledge is a human activity, this action is based on a pre-rational principle that is non-verifiable and therefore non-falsifiable and that marks the starting point of all cognitive, even rational, action. This principle has been given various definitions: metaphysical nucleus (Popper), hard nucleus not subject to test (Lakatos), anterior ideology (Feyerabend), non-dependent paradigm of experience (Kuhn). The rational process is preceded by a pre-rational element, an area of knowledge that cannot be completely investigated rationally and on which attention must be placed due to its problematic, not easily solvable nature.

The discovery of the insurmountable limitations of the scientific method, if not of modernity *tout court,* could be a frustrating task for those faithful to reason, potentially leading to agnostic forms and absolute relativism. On the other hand, within a context that continues to acknowledge the possibility of building general ambits of rationality, these limitations could be exploited as possible resources. A radical way of addressing the pre-rational element that leads to scientific knowledge is, for example, to highlight the value of metaphoric knowledge in science (Kuhn), which paves the way for theories that embrace modalities of knowledge generally considered typical of art. On this issue I point out the argument, provocative only in appearance, according to which certain methods of artistic expression are largely based on rational and knowledge procedures, while methods of scientific discovery in certain instances stem from factors such as imagination, sensibility, emotion, chance-taking, etc.—traits normally attributed to artistic creations (Feyerabend). In this way one is urged to acknowledge the validity of significant forms of knowledge that in a relationship of reciprocal integration equate rational knowledge with other types of discoveries in a trans-disciplinary approach that transverses and transcends scientific disciplines. In this sense it is not enough to adopt an interdisciplinary approach that aims to integrate various specific disciplinary contributions by applying definite methodologies. The complexity of the world requires a transdisciplinary outlook that is capable of creating omnidirectional interactions, starting from specific problematic situations, and establishing exchanges of feedback between the scientific world and the methods of knowledge specific to other fields. This process requires curiosity, will, and sensibility and is a step toward Steiner's vision of cognitive processes.

Personally, I have always instinctively understood knowledge in this sense. In my attempts to understand the hidden secrets of certain ambits of nature, I have continuously sought connections and relations, adopting various points of view and pursuing diverging paths when faced with problems or challenges. I have tried as much as possible to gain an overall outlook and pinpoint the crux of the problem before me. In this sense I have been slightly generalist by widening my knowledge in different fields and directions, sometimes even sacrificing specialist aspects. Maybe emotionally I feel the coldness that is inherent to specialist and technical matters, so that instinctively I try to capture only those aspects that I need to increase my knowledge. This has no doubt been the cause of my anxiety of sorts. Psychologically I would feel more at ease if I could master certain techniques of medical practice. From this viewpoint, I have always admired my surgeon colleagues who are able to perform delicate and complicated surgeries and save human lives. At one time I had good dexterity, which I could have put to good use and improved, but emotionally I was drawn toward another direction so that in fact I have never considered the possibility of nurturing this ability. I have come to terms with my anxiety, accepting it as a natural consequence of acquiring knowledge. The more you know, the more you realize your limitations in grasping the complexity of the world. By trying to continuously find points of juncture between different fields of knowledge I have avoided the risk of considering the experimental data I have collected (for example, on cancer research) as an absolute truth. This way I have always been aware that what I was looking for in the single experiments were data deriving from a simplification of reality.

This simplification is necessary in scientific research in order to control various experimental parameters and to evaluate any variations and repetitions over time. Simplification or reduction must not, however, lead us to mistaken conclusions that do not fall within the context of the data.

Nowadays, at a point when scientific research is making essential contributions thanks to experimental reduction and to the awesome mass of information available to us, we are too often bombarded with astounding declarations. Not a day goes by that you don't hear about the discovery (at experimental level) of a new gene that apparently has been found to play a fundamental role in causing or, as the case may be, fighting cancer. This specially conceived weapon inhibits or encourages the gene's expression and presumably serves as a fundamental means of fighting cancer. Unfortunately, we know that this is not reality. As we have said before, tumorous diseases arise from serious alterations of multiple genes and are the result of an imbalance of the epigenetic code in an embryonic sense. To think of fighting cancer by changing the expression of a single gene or by inserting a healthy gene in the place of a mutated one is truly oversimplifying, not to mention misleading.

Even worse is when discoveries are hailed as groundbreaking, with claims that certain individual characteristics, which usually depend on a series of factors, multiple genes, and the environment, are due to a single gene. The media inundates us with stories of single genes that have been found to be responsible for homosexuality, intelligence, thrill-seeking, and so on. Thank goodness these discoveries sink into oblivion after in-depth analysis proves the utter inconsistency of these claims. Indeed, it is extremely rare that the association between a gene and a personality trait is so simple. Even in the field of pathology, diseases in which the alteration of a single gene leads to a variation of the phenotype are extremely rare. In fact, less than two percent of all diseases are due to the alteration of a single gene. In the remaining ninety-eight percent of gene-related pathologies the presence or absence of disease and its level of gravity are linked to the expression of multiple genes and the environment. It is simpler to study diseases brought on by the alteration of a single gene, and so many researchers analyze the relationships between genes and disease, basing their work on the small minority of pathologies in which one gene is responsible for change in the phenotype.

It is a popular misconception that genes directly and discretely determine an individual's aspect and behavior. The individual is considered to be virtually at the mercy of a highly sophisticated machine manipulated by his or her genes. A similar view of the way genes work is based on the belief, in no small measure fueled by economic powers with a strong vested interest, that biotechnology will give geneticists unlimited powers. Geneticists are viewed as magicians capable of manipulating the code of life and changing it as they please by correcting all of the code's errors. This misconception is based on the belief that the causal relationship between genes and personality (expression of characteristics) is simple and predictable, and that together identical genes can produce inevitably identical phenotypes. Not only is this misconception entirely off base, it is damaging. We cannot exclude the possibility that in the future some doctors or geneticists will make people believe that they can change the fate of an embryo simply by manipulating its DNA. Ideally this will not happen. Despite the media's obsession, it is unlikely that predictive medicine based on presumptions—an activity currently more comparable to astrology than to an exact science—will obtain the results hoped for.

Uncontrollable factors are continuously at play that can change events. We could sequence an individual's entire genome, but the interrelations between heredity and environment are so complex that we cannot simply sum the total of their average effects and from that sum predict an individual's strong and weak points. A given gene does not lead to a given phenotype.

Biologists have known for some time that all multicellular beings, including humans, are highly plastic in terms of their development. To attempt to predict a phenotype based on the genotype, we have to consider too that it is possible for two or more different genomes to give rise to identical phenotypes. Irrespective of genetic and environmental differences, certain aspects of the phenotype seem to have significant stability. On the one side it is therefore possible to have identical genes that lead to very different phenotypes, and on the other different genes that produce like phenotypes. The extent of the complexity of the interrelation among genes was made clear after geneticists started to use genetic engineering to deactivate or "knock out" certain genes. To their surprise they discovered that silencing genes, a process that was deemed to play an important role in certain stages of development, had no influential effect. The final phenotype remained exactly the same. Somehow the genome is able to compensate for the missing gene. This happens because there is a structural and functional redundancy underlying the genome that renders many gene deformities irrelevant for the phenotype. The network of interaction at the basis of life is such that it can compensate and adapt to a myriad of genetic and environmental changes. If this were not possible, maybe life would not be possible. We exist because we are constantly able to adapt. We must change continuously in order to remain stable and maintain our internal equilibrium.

Clearly, scientific reductionism is not able to completely capture the biological reality that makes life possible. We risk being misled and taken down a wrong and dangerous road. In tumorous diseases, reductionism hinders understanding of the complexity of phenomena.

To more deeply understand tumorous diseases one needs to overcome the paradigm of reductionism and focus on complexity. It is evident that even reductive studies using single molecules are relatively pertinent to the context in which the molecules are used. Likewise, an embryonic growth factor behaves as such in a given context, but behaves as a differentiation factor in a different context. As I have already mentioned, many molecules are two-faced. In the same embryo are processes that on one side create life and on the other create death. Death plays a key role in creating the embryo. For instance, programmed cell death gives rise to arms, legs, hands, and feet. Initially, an embryo has webbed hands. Then, signals issued by neighboring cells lead to the programmed cellular death (apoptosis) of the tissue that unites the fingers so that they can be separate. Mammals and land birds have separate fingers and toes, while aquatic mammals and birds have webbed fingers and toes. This could mean that the processes that control apoptosis might have played a pivotal role in evolution, and that the death mechanisms are the fruit of the evolutionary processes.

Asexual organisms are essentially immortal since they duplicate in identical forms. Death appears in sexual organisms with the loss of replicate units and with the appearance of differentiation processes. Tumor cells are immortal because they have lost the ability to differentiate and can only replicate. If embryos were not able to differentiate and install cell life and death programs, they would become giant tumors. In very rare cases, embryos that are unable to install apoptosis programs turn into malignant tumors called vesicular mole, made up of immortalized cells that metastasize. This happens when on the one hand the embryo has not acquired the ability to correct genetic damage arising from environmental or hereditary defects, and on the other the mother is unable to produce the molecule that protects the life of the embryo.

In our labs, we studied the apoptosis control mechanisms present in embryos, such as the p53 oncosuppressor (the "guardian of babies"), as well as the maternal control on the life of the embryo by isolating in the pregnant uterine mucus a fraction of 10 kDaltons that we have called the "Life-Protecting Factor." Through this factor the mother protects the life of the embryo by killing pathological cell clones such as aggressive tumors or dangerous clones. Luckily vesicular mole is a rare tumor in which both the mother and the embryo are altered. Life uses significant measures to arise!

At this point, it should be clear that studies on single genes, single receptors, or single-action mechanisms should be taken relatively, while more attention should be focused on studies of context and relations. Studies on differentiation processes have now led to a complexity model in which robust biological networks and not a linear information process leads stem cells to conformational landscapes that increasingly channel them toward definitive differentiation.

This concept emerged as early as the 1940s when the English embryologist and geneticist Conrad Waddington painted the processes of embryo development and differentiation as an "epigenetic landscape" made of hills and valleys through which fertilized egg cells channel in subsequent divisions and differentiations until they become liver cells, kidney cells, brain cells, etc., and therefore make up an entire organism. To organize itself life must follow fairly straightforward paths and not a linear and infinite series of punctual information. If this were not the case, life would not exist on this planet. Even the smallest mistakes would be enough to render the program ineffective.

Luckily, organisms follow various rules to arise and maintain balance. These rules are the outcome of a natural restriction imposed by the formation of the regulatory epigenetic network and the underlying genetic network. Life is a continuous flow of molecules and energy in which the information-rich structure of the context, the network's qualitative and quantitative composition, takes precedence over the single molecule. A single molecule, just like a single bit, provides very little information. The composition of such networks is important and makes up the "attractor" landscape through which stem cells create life.

The concept of an attractor landscape is referred to in fractal mathematics and the chaos theory and sums up the behavior of stem cells and biology in an organism. This does not mean that detailed information on aspects of specific molecules should be overlooked. It is important, but it should be taken in context. Studies on, say, a leaf cannot be expected to apply to the entire forest; even less so can it be expected that by modifying a leaf the entire forest is therefore modified. And yet this is exactly what simplification leads us to believe. The discovery of an important gene in cancer genesis does not mean that a cure for cancer is just around the corner.

Fortunately, studies have progressed and led us farther and farther away from these illusions. However, it seems as though excessively high hopes are being raised on the use of stem cells, this likely because large economic interests are at stake. Based on these false hopes, people without scruples are committing crimes in order to get their hands on stem cells; we read it in the newspapers every day. Not only are these criminal acts despicable, they are pointless and stupid.

To understand the reach of this problem, we must overcome this simplistic view and rely on other scientific paradigms. I refer to studies on contexts and the relationships that exist among various entities. The scientific paradigm, which has as its purpose research on the relationship among the various entities and contexts within which they act, is that of complexity. It is from the study of these complex adaptive systems that models have emerged and explained very well how, for example, our metabolic network is composed. This particular model explains how the metabolic network is made up of a network of small worlds. The organization of these networks is by no means limited to biology but can be found in society and ecology. A few years ago the sociologist Duncan J. Watts[3] spoke at a conference held in Milan and attended by the Nobel Prize winner Murray Gell-Mann. Watts explained how these networks of small worlds apply to society. On Earth all of us are connected by "six degrees of separation." It emerged from the conference that the networks likely represent one of the important methods through which life is organized in all its various aspects. Transportation networks, airport hubs, and Internet search engines all function on the same concept. The large Internet search engines were the first to understand the importance of the hub concept.

The networks of life in general are networks of small worlds whereby at metabolic level they signify a modular organization.

Each module (which is a part of the network) is usually made up of several components and is characterized by its own functional meaning. There is a module for protein synthesis, one for metabolizing carbohydrates, one for metabolizing cholesterol or triglycerides, and so on. Each module is relatively isolated so that it can avoid any damage that might affect other modules and is able to self-repair. Each module is also sufficiently linked to the rest to know if and when to enter into action. Basically, each module is linked to other modules through "nodes" or substances that are shared by several modules. In this way information can easily flow between the modules with linked nodes. The molecules linked to the main node can easily link up with other molecules that are part of a different module. The different modules are then grouped in a hierarchy that ends up including the entire metabolism.

A similar modular system organized in networks also exists inside the cell where, as I mentioned earlier, the genes communicate and "speak" to one another. Such a system is highly resilient and able to respond to any damage flexibly and economically, thereby maintaining functional integrity even in the event of widespread damage. Living organisms are usually able to repair damage due to disease and environmental aggressions precisely because they have the amazing ability to regulate and are adaptable and resilient. Although they are organized by modules, they work as a single cognitive network by virtue of essential nodes of communication that interlink the entire system and very rapidly exchange messages.

In light of the above, it is clear that when such a network is seriously altered, as in the case of tumorous diseases, it is no longer enough to repair just one point; rather, multiple levels must be repaired in order to correct the main ruptures. In this way, the network can complete the process through its reacquired ability to self-repair.

It is therefore evident why reductionism poses so many limitations in understanding tumorous diseases. It is not possible to understand and intervene on the process in one single point of the network and thus this reductive approach is extremely restrictive in adopting effective therapeutic strategies. Only destructive and, unfortunately, toxic therapies can be applied through simplification. Indeed, it is difficult to apply the reductive paradigm to regulation and differentiation therapies that "teach" tumor cells how to change and not be aggressive. At this point I will explain why this is so.

Although reductionism has been superseded as a reference model, it is still widely used in the scientific field and, more importantly, in the economic field, in particular the pharmaceutical industry. This paradigm has led research all over the world to focus only on punctual mechanisms and punctual studies of single molecules. As a result, this approach has affected Health Ministries the world over and their legislation on drug authorization. Pharmaceutical companies have heavily exploited this concept and outlook and taken it to extreme consequences, in no small part for competition reasons. The legislation of the Health Ministries in countries around the world has become increasingly restrictive, often instituting very restrictive and punctual procedures. This has adversely affected the pharmaceutical segment at global level so that given the astronomical costs that such procedures entail, pharmaceutical giants are the only ones able to withstand the clearance of new drugs. Large pharmaceutical groups have thus done away with smaller competitors. The company restructurings that have taken place since the 1970s have in fact eliminated all small- and medium-sized companies and obligated the large corporations to merge, leaving the world drug market in the hands of a few.

Today these giant corporations are caught in a paradoxical situation. Although they have accumulated huge fortunes, they are cornered by inflexible drug legislation mechanisms (which they in no small part helped to create) and limited in creating innovations that today could be revolutionary. If we take the example of tumorous diseases, the strategy of these corporations seems to center on identifying more accurate weapons, or "intelligent" bullets to hit the cancer cells that they single out and target. Progress has been made in the form of "intelligent weapons" such as monoclonal antibodies, cell cycle inhibitors, angiogenesis inhibitors, and proteasome inhibitors. However, it should be noted that these weapons may be toxic and are effective only against certain types of cancer. Moreover, as I will explain in detail in Chapter 9, tumor cells are "intelligent" cells that learn to defend themselves when under attack. After repeated treatment cycles, tumor cells become resistant to attack, and unless the tumor has been completely destroyed down to the last cell, it can reform and expand even more aggressively than before. Conversely, in differentiation therapy, cells are "educated" and taught to behave correctly and to differentiate or die spontaneously, thereby avoiding any war-like confrontation or the effects of resistance.

Unfortunately, this vision clashes with the interests of today's pharmaceutical industry, interests that obviously play a major role in determining the direction of scientific research. What's more, this has become an unintentional, almost subconscious act on the part of pharmaceutical companies that today function as part of a self-propelled mechanism that's virtually impossible to reverse or supersede. It's not true that pharmaceutical companies do not want scientific progress. They probably do, but they have become a prisoner of the paradigm that prohibits them from making any substantial progress. This key question must be pondered and resolved if we all are to avoid being trapped. We must find solutions that can introduce substantial changes in how we perceive current medical therapy, not just in the oncological field, but also in regard to other pathologies. These changes should give us the tools to shift from therapies centered on synthesis molecules that do not repair the organism and have adverse effects, to therapy using networks of biological molecules that constitute a correct information therapy aimed at balancing the networks of which the organism is made.

The era of synthesis chemistry is ending in medicine, to make way for increasingly effective biological therapies. This is the only road open to regenerative stem-cell therapies. The day will come when it will be understood that only by using specific networks of differentiation factors or growth factors will we be able to control the pathways toward cell differentiation or toward expansion.

Unless we start from this point, the fight against cancer and degenerative diseases in general will achieve limited results. Nature provides us with means that as needed give into or modify nature. Specific differentiation networks could be vital in cancer therapy. Today, however, the only cancer therapies that have been tested are based on the concept of tumor destruction. For many years science has proceeded along this path, and this must be acknowledged. This is the situation and it is pointless to deny it. Therapy data show the consolidated effectiveness of chemotherapy and radiotherapy, and for now we cannot think otherwise. What we can do at this stage is create an association between traditional therapies and modulation and differentiation therapies. Among other things, our results obtained in the lab experiments conducted at the Sapienza University in Rome show that there is a synergistic effect in the association between some chemotherapeutic agents and stem-cell differentiation factors. In at least some types of cancer, like colon cancer, this has become evident. In the meantime, while we wait for further improvement in the effectiveness of the exclusive use of differentiation factors, this association could be a possible solution for now. In the future, as research develops, increasingly effective therapies aimed at normalizing tumor cells could be created. At experimental level, it has been proven that differentiation factors of stem cells are able to normalize tumor cells by making them lose their malignant behavior.

When our experiments demonstrated that tumor cells can re-differentiate themselves, I asked myself why the modification of the epigenetic and genetic code in terms of differentiation could be so important in determining a tumor cell's more benign behavior. This question was critical in order to proceed to further and to more deeply understanding biological phenomena. As soon as I asked myself this question I realized that a fundamental problem lay before me that I could have addressed a long time ago. But questions arise when they want to and when we are ready to accept them. I realized that I was back in a familiar situation. My mind started working overtime, and I became obsessed with this question. I struggled to keep my wits about me and keep the problem at arm's length. I tried to find rational and scientific answers. I would tell myself that, unlike stem cells, differentiated cells deactivated most multiplication genes and that was no doubt why they did not multiply and were not aggressive. This answer did not satisfy me in the least. I realized that this explanation was centered on molecular mechanisms and only scratched the surface of the problem. Underneath there had to be more, something more profound. But what? I had to find out. Seeing as I was no longer able to get the question and the problem out of my head, I hoped the answer would come to me quickly.

Chapter 9

Information and Consciousness

"Cells communicate with one another by using codes of meaning."

At 5 a.m. one summer morning I suddenly awoke with this phrase branded in my mind. In fact I think I woke up precisely because that phrase had entered my mind as I was sleeping.

It was a beautiful day. The air was still cool and you could already see the light of the sun beginning to dawn. As soon as I woke up I was filled with energy and ready to tackle the thoughts that were crowding my mind.

I don't know exactly how this happened because I never wake up before 7 a.m., and when I do it takes me a while before I make contact with reality. I move about sleepily and need the jolt of a few cups of coffee before I can get my brain to function. That morning I didn't need any of this. I felt refreshed and ready to start thinking.

What was the meaning of the sentence "Cells communicate with one another by using codes of meaning"? Perhaps it meant that cells understand the meaning of messages and are thus intelligent? If this were true that phrase obviously had to be understood in a literal and not a metaphorical sense. In this case, the issue before me would be hard to explain and resolve. To say that a cell has the ability to understand the meaning of a message is the same as saying that molecules and all the factors of the microenvironment that surround it carry information, and that cells process this information, decode, integrate, and understand it not only in form but also in terms of message content. These messages therefore elicit responses that relay information to all the other cells nearby or far away on the content of the processing and on any other messages that might need to be transmitted.

But how could I prove this? A thought flashed through my mind: maybe I could try to find a solution by tapping into the knowledge

I had gained as an occupational physician in the field of toxicology. After all, I had taught toxicology at the specialization school in occupational medicine at the University of Trieste, and therefore I could at least try to unravel the enigma that lay before me.

The question at the root of the problem was the following: when coming into contact for the first time with a new and unknown substance, how does a cell know, for instance, if that substance is toxic or not? A toxic agent does not carry a label that reads "I am toxic."

I realized that answering that question would be virtually impossible if I considered cells as isolated systems, but the endeavor became possible if instead I saw cells as being a part of the context of a complex adaptive system autonomous from, but communicating with, its surrounding environment.

My task therefore became to track the fate of a substance located inside a complex system, such as an organism, that for the first time comes into contact with a cell. Let's say that this molecule, in relation to which the organism has no idea how to behave or which metabolic paths to pursue, gives rise to toxic effects. The liver is usually the organ entrusted with detoxification, and when facing this substance for the first time it is capable of not only assimilating the form of the substance but also understanding the content of the message. If the substance is toxic, the liver cells put a system of detoxification into motion and if necessary will modify themselves to speed up biotransformative processes that turn a toxic substance into a harmless one. How is this possible?

It is possible because the complete cell differentiation process, which gives rise to a new being, identifies with the emerging of the mind and the cognitive process. This affects the brain, which is the specific structure through which the cognitive process acts. It is the organism as a whole with all of its subsystems and organs that works as a single cognitive network. It is the emergence of this organismic identity, of a new complex adaptive system, that renders the subsystems capable of understanding the meaning of a message. In other words, when a new being is formed, the regulation and control system of each cell not only governs the cell in question, it links up with all the systems of the other cells. This surprising level of coherency that is established from the very start of embryonic development is what makes life possible. This occurs in all animal species when a new identity is formed, a unit that functions as an organism. When an organism with its own individuality is formed, the characteristics that complexity researchers attribute to complex adaptive systems arise. A complex adaptive system has the capacity to: a) learn from experience; b) generate new self-similar systems; and c) perceive information as a flow of data, codify it, and express it as a "scheme."

It is this complex capacity that sets an organism apart from a group of cells. The organism is much more than the sum of its parts precisely because of its abilities acquired through the system and cognitive network organization. Returning to the example of the liver cell, it should be noted that if a liver cell is decontextualized and put *in vitro,* it cannot "understand" the "meaning" of toxicity, as it has no links with the network that provides all the information useful for signification. The organismic network informs the liver cell that the molecule is "toxic."

In terms of toxicology, a molecule is deemed toxic when it is able to cause damage to different organs based on its tropism, or to the entire organism if it has systemic effects. As a consequence of the damage, various molecules are produced that are not present in physiological conditions and are indeed the expression of the damage. For instance, if a substance is irritating and causes inflammatory processes, the organism will contain many of the substances that are usually produced in these cases; or if the substance causes necrosis, the circulatory flow will contain various molecules that are the expression of cell death. When these molecules reach the liver cell, this latter records the presence of the substance, integrates the various signals, and understands that this foreign substance is causing damage. When the liver cell comes into contact with a foreign substance, even for the first time, it knows that it has to direct it to metabolic pathways that will deprive it of its toxicity. In essence, the liver cell (or any other cell within the organism) has many options. It chooses from among these options based on the information that it processes and receives from the organism (understood as a cognitive network). If the cell were not contextualized, the organism would not receive any information from the network, and because it would not know which option to choose, it would be killed by the toxic molecule. This explains why decontextualized cells die easily, and why those within the network resist attack and are so resilient. The organism makes the single cell intelligent and able to send and understand messages. The context is the key. It is the context that ensures that the various chemical or chemical-physical reactions occurring are not the expression of simple mechanical events or blind determinism. The context directs the information and ensures different behavior from the same molecule. I mentioned earlier that in certain contexts an embryonic factor can give rise to multiplication, while in others it can give rise to differentiation.

At biological level, there are different levels of freedom of choice, and these determine intelligent behavior aimed at maintaining life. Life and information are indivisibly connected. Information and intelligent behavior are one and the same, at all levels of life. We must therefore admit that a certain type of cognition is deeply incarnated and that the entire process, which also includes perception and behavior, is one of the intrinsic characteristics of living systems. A living system is characterized by the fact that it can change continuously and yet maintain the reticular structure of organization. All living organisms renew themselves uninterruptedly as their cells, which are undergoing continuous metabolic processes, demolish and build structures, tissues, and organs and replace the damaged cells. And yet the organism retains its identity, its scheme of organization. A living system structurally adapts in an intelligent manner to its environment by continuously interacting with it, and each interaction triggers continuous changes within the organism. The structural changes modify the future behavior of the living system. My point is that a living being is a system that learns. This type of learning does not necessarily require the existence of a brain or even a nervous system. Because they constantly adapt to the environment we can say that all living beings are intelligent. All living beings learn the various paths of adaptation to the environment through their history as an individual and as a species. As a result, living beings are constantly changing their structure, leaving traces of themselves and their prior development. These structural changes affect future behavior. Consequently, we can say that the behavior of every living organism is determined by its structural network. Humberto Maturana and Francisco Varela, founders of the Santiago theory of cognition, maintain that cognition is tightly linked to self-poiesis (the ability of living networks to self-regenerate). A system is self-poietic when it continuously undergoes structural changes but at the same time keeps its reticular model of organization. It not only specifies by itself its structural changes, it also specifies which stimuli from the environment should activate these changes. Basically, a living system retains the freedom to decide which stimuli deserve attention and, if the stimuli are capable of causing disturbance, which ones should be avoided. In this sense, the structural changes within living systems are, according to the Santiago theory, cognitive acts. A living system interacts cognitively with its environment. The life process itself is a cognitive process. Development and learning are two faces of the same coin.

This concept sheds new light on the age-old question of freedom and determinism. But because the behavior of a living organism depends on its structure, we can say that it is both determined and free. The behavior of a living organism has various degrees of freedom, all of which are determined by the organism's structure.

With incredible intuition author Umberto Eco, although not a biologist, in 1990 at a symposium entitled "The Semiotics of Cellular Communication" stated that:

> It is not necessary to oppose a high behavior (human) against a low behavior (biological). It is sufficient to refer to two abstract models: i) a triadic model where between A and B there is an unpredictable and potentially infinite series of Cs; and ii) a dyadic model in which A provokes B without any mediation. There is a space of choice and supposed indetermination, while the non-space between A and B is a non-space of blind necessity and of inevitable determination. Many human questions are governed by this second model. I do not find it difficult to accept the idea that many biological processes are governed by the first model, that is if it can be proven.[4]

In light of the above, I think that the proof of a space of freedom at biological level has already been sufficiently demonstrated. In this space of freedom, cells, at organismic level, communicate intelligently, with each cell adapting to the needs of the other. This happens by virtue of the fact that the genetic and epigenetic codes, even given their plasticity, use the same scheme to decode and interpret messages. These codes are modulated during embryogenesis, regulated differently in each differentiated cell, but in each cell the codes have maintained the same tuning and the same capability to signify the messages. An example of a higher communication level in life is during pregnancy when two beings collaborate and renew life.

As I have already stated, our lab studies demonstrated that during pregnancy the mother cooperates decisively in embryonic development and that the uterus is not a mechanical container; it is a regulating organ. More specifically, in our lab tests we isolated from the pregnant uterine mucous membrane of several mammals a low-molecular-weight fraction, less than 10 kDaltons, able to inhibit the growth of various types of *in vitro* tumors, inducing in the tumor cells a metabolic path that leads to programmed cellular death. This fraction is already present in the pregnant uterine mucous membrane when the fertilized egg is implanted, well before the organs and systems of the embryo are formed, including the brain. The fraction is inactive on normal cells but seems to be able to identify and destroy any cell that does not undergo normal development and/or threatens the life of the embryo, be it a tumor cell or an activated lymphocyte. We therefore termed this fraction the "Life-Protecting Factor" to signify the cross-talk that takes place between mother and child and in which, even if the signifiers are not sound waves but traces of molecules, the meanings are clearly communicated nonetheless.

We are not able to pick up on this communication, which occurs at all levels of the universe, because we have an intrinsic limitation—our mind, which is able to grasp only certain realities. Reality as we know it through our studies and experimental methods of simplification is only a small part of the reality surrounding us, which is much richer and more complex.

For this reason, we must be modest and cautious in making certain claims, as it is a well-known fact that the deeper we delve into knowledge, the clearer our limitations as humans become. Often we do not take into account these limitations, and we make declarations that are obsolete as soon as they are uttered.

Returning to the discussion on life and meaning—the embryo and communication at the level of living beings—a heated debate has arisen recently among illustrious members of the scientific community on the claim of some scientists that an embryo can be considered a human being only when the organs and systems are formed, more specifically the brain. This affirmation was presumably based on simplistic observation, which attributes all cognitive functions to the brain (on the basis of which human beings are distinguished from groups of cells that have not yet been characterized as an individual). This has been an extremely difficult and often controversial debate, especially in regard to the use of embryonic stem cells for research purposes. In Italy, before a referendum was held, embryonic stem cell research involved the destruction of embryos in formation. Currently, we are trying to prevent this from happening, even though the results of various researches underway are not yet clear. The affirmations of important exponents of research were supposed to confirm the scientific grounds of this issue. However, as I mentioned earlier, reality is much more complex than we think. What we thought was only a group of stem cells without meaning, in reality, after in-depth study, turned out to be something entirely different. These cells are an "emerging reality," a new being of which the mother is aware. Not, as we mentioned earlier, in a metaphoric sense, but in a literal sense. The mother protects this new being, which she recognizes as an individual other than herself that needs to be protected and preserved. The dialogue between mother and embryo is necessary in order to organize life. When this cross-talk is interrupted, life is threatened. We already saw how when the mother is not able to produce the protective molecules and the embryo undergoes damage that it does not know how to repair, the pregnancy becomes a malignant tumor called vesicular mole. Whenever communication is cut off among the cells of an organism, life is in danger. The same happens when a person falls ill with cancer.

In a cancer patient the dialogue between the individual and a group of cells is interrupted. These cells are part of a subgroup that has developed, and its codes of signification have become different from those used by all the other differentiated cells in the organism to communicate. These codes are linked to one of the possible configurations present in the stage of embryonic undifferentiation and belong to a complex adaptive system (the embryo) in which the basic message is to "organize life." This is how a tumor cell organizes its life, even if this occurs at the expense of the entire organism, of which it is no longer a part. We are confronted with a metalinguistic problem, an incompatibility between codes.[5]

This can explain why differentiated cells cooperate and support each other, while tumor cells are destructive and malignant toward the adult organism. The behavior of tumor cells is a problem that affects not only the cell and its genes.

For this reason an explanation based solely on molecular mechanisms that view the process as being a result of the activity of genes and growth factors, which push neoplastic cells toward continuous multiplication, did not fully satisfy me and made me address the problem in terms of complexity.

Cancer is a complex adaptive system that tries to self-organize: progression, the formation of new blood vessels, remote metastasis are all the evolutionary steps of a complex system that attempts to create life at all costs. This complexity, however, has not been easy to grasp and identify. I think it was useful for us to reflect on the methods of communication in living systems, as in this way it has been possible to demonstrate what reductionism cannot understand at the biological level: the relationship between entities within a context, the methods of communication in living systems, and the problems stemming from incompatibility among codes. The behavior of tumor cells derives precisely from this incompatibility in that the tumor cell is not a part of the adult organism but rather evolves as an autonomous entity, a new complex adaptive system. Only contact with "its own" embryonic microenvironment can reinstate communication. At embryonic level, the differentiation networks must be found so that the dialogue between tumor and diseased individual can flow. Indeed, specific differentiation networks must be identified for each disease. The way has been paved; we must now do what it takes to follow it to the end.

Cancer is the most serious communication pathology. Cancer is to the body as psychosis is to the mind. Both pathologies destroy the integrity of the mind-body adaptive system, in other words, the organism. Matter and consciousness are inextricably bound to one another, even though consciousness as such emerges as a "new reality" in complex living organisms, such as humans. Consciousness, or experience through awareness, is a more limited phenomenon than cognition, which affects all levels of life. Inner experience appears progressively in the evolution of animal behavior and expresses itself in its most complex form in humans. It is the result of a series of emerging abilities that are able to open up a qualitatively different world. This world is governed by its own laws and is autonomous from the material world, even though the two are tightly connected and influence each other. The same is true in the relationship between the world of life, which also manifests itself following large emerging abilities, and the world of non-living matter. Growing levels of complexity give rise to emerging abilities and, in the case of consciousness, these levels of complexity are reached through highly evolved development.

As the situation now stands, there seems to be agreement to some extent among scholars of consciousness in distinguishing two types of cognitive experience that emerge at different levels of complexity. The first type, "primary consciousness," occurs when the cognitive process is accompanied by a basic perceptive and emotional experience. Most animals seem to possess this type of consciousness. The second type, which includes self-consciousness, is known as "reflexive consciousness." From this latter type of consciousness we formulate beliefs, values, and strategies; it emerges through language, the inner world of concepts, and ideas that create cultural phenomena and organized social relationships.

Today there are many branches of study on consciousness. I will limit myself to mentioning the main branches, from the one defined by Francisco Varela as neuroreductionist, of which a prominent figure is Francis Crick (winner, together with James Watson, of the Nobel Prize for their discovery of the double-helix structure of

DNA; Crick maintains that consciousness is reduced to the activity of neurons and makes up an emerging ability of the brain *in toto*), to functionalism (according to which states of consciousness are defined by their "functional organization" and can therefore be understood provided their scheme of organization has been identified; there are multiple variations on this branch, with many proposed schemes of organization of states of consciousness), to neurophenomenology (a hybrid methodology that combines neuroscience with phenomenological philosophy to study consciousness). All these schools share the notion that consciousness is a cognitive process that emerges from complex neural activity. However, others, mostly physicists and mathematicians, advocate the idea that consciousness is an ability that stems from matter rather than from the mind. The mathematician Roger Penrose claims that consciousness is the expression of quantum gravity, something we could understand better if we understood the physical world better.

In my opinion, none of these efforts or current studies on functional neuroimaging (attempts to discover what's inside the "black box" of the human brain) or investigations, even those able to discover the "dance of quantum particles or atoms" in the brain, can solve the mystery of consciousness.

The problem of consciousness is even more complex. It is linked to sub-consciousness, without us being aware of it. The sub-consciousness structures and molds all our conscious thought. In turn, sub-consciousness is a reality resulting from our body, in which instincts, sensations, and emotions intermingle with thoughts and cognitive acts. Our consciousness is profoundly incarnated, bound and modeled by our sub-consciousness and corporeal experience. For instance, we perceive space in a certain way because our body has a specific dimension, and through our body we project this dimension onto other objects. Our body, in other words, acts as a benchmark in our relationship with space and guides us in establishing relationships between objects. We use our body to construct mental images through which we are able to conceive abstract categories. Our consciousness is thus tightly bound to our body, and thought is partly determined by the sub-conscious. Although incarnate, consciousness is an emerging reality that differs from and goes beyond the brain and body. It is a reality that somehow transcends and self-informs the nervous system and the rest of the body. All emerging reality is something more and qualitatively different from the sum of the parts. As I have already mentioned, for every new reality that emerges, a new world emerges. From non-living matter, living matter emerges and from this, on a long evolutionary scale, new forms of life emerge, including forms of conscious and self-conscious life. Evolution therefore gradually brings with it the complete expression of unexpressed potential present from the beginning. Within this context and from this perspective, we can conclude that matter, life, and consciousness must have existed unexpressed from the very beginning. These notions, though compatible with an interpretative theory of evolution, known as "constructive theory of evolution," clash violently with Darwinism and neo-Darwinism. Natural selection is based on chance and necessity and is the cornerstone of Darwin's theory. Today, this theory is held to be inadequate in explaining the course of discontinuous evolution that constitutes the history of this world.[6]

New evolutions with emerging abilities may be explained instead through processes of constructive interaction in which two or more entities unite and cooperate, determining through their integration new and unpredictable qualities. The creation of complex adaptive systems within this context can be seen as based on interactions that on the one side can be linked to matter with regard to forces and energy, but also, on the other side, as an intangible reality in terms of information and organizational intelligence. In addition to biologists, who are struggling to lay the foundation of an evolutionary theory based on constructive cooperation, other scholars such as Ervin Laszlo[7] have gone even further by conceiving a fascinating theory whereby all the pieces of current scientific knowledge are composed like a mosaic. For Laszlo, the universe is above all in-formation that connects all things (particles, atoms, molecules, organisms, ecosystems, galaxies, as well as the mind and consciousness associated to these realities) regardless of the distance in space and time. Behind the increase in complexity due to evolutionary events, coherent processes of in-formation exist and ensure the cooperative behavior of all the components of the system (this concept seems to echo the system of "implicated order" of David Bohm) until the emergence of individual and collective consciousness. The cosmic vacuum, though lacking matter, is in fact no vacuum but is the site of this in-formation, from which everything is generated. The quantum vacuum, also defined as the "Akashic field" (in Sanskrit *Akasha* means "space" from which everything originates), is not only the source from which everything originates, including new universes, it is also a kind of cosmic memory, a virtually infinite database in which every event in the universe leaves its trace, thereby determining subsequent evolutions. Individual human consciousness is therefore no longer considered a reality isolated from the organism; rather, it is intimately connected to the universe of which it is a part.

Reductionists will be shocked by these conclusions and thus will turn a blind eye in an attempt to close a debate that poses a great danger to them. Clearly, for those such as molecular biologists, who view life as a series of molecules and chemical reactions, a systemic vision according to which life arises out of organized structures and relationships and that even goes so far as to entertain the possibility that intelligence and consciousness self-inform these structures poses a potentially destructive debate that must be avoided at all costs. Yet it is becoming increasingly clear that what we once considered a single structure of the universe, visible matter, is a miniscule part of the universe, which, more than likely, as a whole, is largely information and intelligence. Visible matter accounts for only four percent of the universe, while twenty-one percent is dark matter, the first 3D map of which has just recently been made, and seventy-five percent dark energy, i.e., energy of which we know nothing except that it is responsible for the ever rapidly expanding universe. In an attempt to unify all the forces of nature and conceive a "theory of everything" that coherently explains the origin and physics of the universe, physical theorists are discovering hidden dimensions. Thus we have string theories (single ultramicroscopic units immersed in the profoundness of matter and rolled up in the folds of space and whose modes of vibration determine the intimate constitution of matter); the theory of the multiverse (which generates other universes); and the holographic theory (according to which the universe is a mere interpretation of our brain from light waves and appears as a 3D image, but in reality is a super hologram in which the past, present, and future co-exist simultaneously and in which the quantum vacuum is the origin of the information and intelligence that links everything instantaneously).

Of course, these are only theories and have yet to be verified. We do not know which of these or others that I have not mentioned or theories not formulated yet will be the most suitable to explain the nature of the universe. However, the mere fact that these theories exist shows that what we see and perceive is only a small part of reality. The heavens harbor great complexity that can only be beneficial in fighting fundamentalism and dogmatism.

Explaining reality merely on the basis of what we can see and subject to experiment is presumptuous and limiting. Indeed, we must test, verify, and falsify as much as possible, but we also have to admit that other realities exist even if we cannot understand them or completely verify them. Consciousness and intelligence are a reality present within us and most likely in the universe.

One day, perhaps, we will better understand how this intelligence characterized and *self-informed* the entire universe. To the coldness of rationality and fact-finding activities we must add the warmth of sentiment and willingness. This would allow us to see many more things than cold reason alone allows us to see. The poets know this and can thus reach illuminating conclusions. Returning to the issue of life and knowledge, Goethe wrote:

> If you want to understand and describe a living being, as a first step you must get rid of its animating principle; then you have in your hands the various parts of it. Only the life bonds will be missing; this is a pity! (*Faust:* "Studierzimmer").

Chapter 10

Stardust

Looking back at the road I have traveled, sometimes I am amazed. I started studying aspects of biology, of single molecules and groups of cells, like those of *in vitro* human tumors, and now, after analyzing the communication methods of living beings, I am presupposing the existence of an intelligence that *self-informs* everything. This surprises me because I never planned to abandon reduction and simplification. Furthermore, I was accustomed to rational processes, proceeding step by step and never taking anything for granted.

Never could I have imagined that my investigations would lead me beyond the behavior of cell groups treated with different molecules. Indeed, my observations on the different levels of responses to treatment shed light on the methods of communication at biological level and led me to consider vaster issues. My thoughts then arose spontaneously and naturally so that I never felt that I had missed any steps of logic. Quite the opposite, everything seemed to me to be interconnected and highly coherent.

What has always puzzled me about basic research—and what I have always considered as being connected to processes of logic that, far from being consequential, are truncated in their evolution—is the mechanical way in which biology and life are viewed. More specifically, these mechanical and deterministic views are acutely accentuated in the vision that genetic engineering has of life.

Because it manipulates "genetic information," genetic engineering has often wrongly been likened to information technology. Unlike this latter, which has undergone a significant revolution thanks to the use of information networks and to the deep understanding of the mechanisms through which information is divulged, genetic engineering has always taken a linear approach and until recently has never taken into account cellular networks, which, as we know, are fundamentally important to biological functions.

In the previous chapters I have harshly criticized genetic determinism, the belief according to which organisms are predictable based on their genetic make-up. As I previously explained, identical genotypes are able to express themselves as completely different phenotypes. Despite this fact, the vision based on genetic determinism is a die-hard one. Today, as I write this, a headline from the Italian newspaper *Sole 24ore*, based on an article in the *International Herald Tribune*, reads:

> Tailor-made dogs in arrival from California. Faster, meaner, more muscular or, on the contrary, slower, less aggressive, more slender. How many of you have at least once complained that your dog was too this or too that? Never again. Thanks to the completion of the first map of a dog genome, you can now have your four-legged friend made to measure. "We're on the verge of a real radical shift in the way we apply genetics in our society," said Mark Neff, associate director of the veterinary genetics laboratory at the University of California. Free of most of the ethical concerns associated with the practice of eugenics in humans, scientists are seizing on new genetic research opportunities in the animal kingdom. Dog breeders are on cloud nine. Now they can create the perfect dog. A superdog with all the options.[8]

Perhaps American dog breeders should take a hard look at certain results before they get their hopes up. I'm afraid they will have to wait a long time and invest heavily in order to achieve the goals they've set. And yet, draining the pockets of those who seek to profit from animal testing would not be such a bad thing. Fortunately, these practices are widely held as inhumane, but even more morally despicable are the people throughout history who have pursued eugenic objectives on humans. Today, it seems these objectives have become more modest so that instead of a "superhuman," we now settle for a "superdog."

Unfortunately, genetic engineering is not limited to experimental lab research. Often the results of this research are used on a wider scale in the market of genetically modified organisms (GMOs) without thorough studies having been conducted on the potential consequences on man and environment. As a result, our ecosystem is suffering real damage.

Applying biotechnology to agriculture is infinitely easier than to animals. Indeed, genetic engineering has achieved some level of success in agriculture precisely because plant cells are relatively simple and, compared to animals, their regulation systems are less sophisticated. It has therefore been possible for geneticists to insert foreign genes into vegetable cells in an attempt to achieve a series of "advantages" that the biotechnology industry has gone to great lengths to publicize: healthier plants tailor-made to meet consumer needs, resistant to insects, herbicides, drought, etc. The industry claims that GMO practices will virtually eliminate the use of pesticides, causing less harm to the environment, yielding bigger and better quality crops, and contributing to the end of world hunger.

First of all, world hunger is not due to a lack of food (food is in overabundance and farmers must often destroy surpluses), but to the fact that food production and distribution is in the hands of the rich and powerful, leaving nothing for the poor. Transgenic seeds have benefited only food manufacturers and not the people who consume them. These seeds are protected under patent and intellectual property law. Biotechnology companies ensure that a farmer's dependency is even greater by making the seeds sterile (through terminator technology) so the patented products must be bought every year. On a wider scale, this practice would be devastating to poor countries. Thus the problem of world hunger would not be solved but on the contrary exacerbated.

Moreover, another risk linked to the use of biotechnology is the skewed view it gives rise to. Basic research is moving toward the artificial modification of the genoma instead of toward processes of regulation and modulation. Research is conducted not to improve health and the quality of life, but to boost profits. Not to mention the environmental risks.

One of the most common biotechnological applications used in farming is aimed at developing herbicide-resistant plants, as I mentioned above. Among the risks in making plants, such as certain types of soy, resistant to herbicides is the fact that these herbicides are then used in increasingly large quantities. One of the most publicized advantages of specific GMOs is resistance to specific herbicides, but this only justifies the use of larger and larger amounts of herbicides to kill weeds. This in turn increases weed resistance to the herbicides. You can see how a vicious cycle is put into motion that leads to even greater uses of herbicides.

The same is true for insect-resistant GMOs. For example, plants modified with a gene extracted from *Bacillus thurigiensis* (Bt gene) have been made able to codify a toxin that kills various insect species. Over time, insect species have evolved resistance to Bt toxin. As a result, we are already witnessing how this is starting to negatively affect the economy and the health of consumers. The large quantities of pesticides and herbicides that are required when the inevitable resistance develops to GMOs will inevitably seep into the food we eat.

Last but not least, we must remember the risk of pollination between transgenic and traditional plants. Genetically modified plants that are not tested for their potential dangers are spreading uncontrollably in the environment and creating risk situations that are not easy to predict. Scientists employed by biotechnology companies usually know little about ecological processes. This is partly because for many years genetic determinism has distorted biology research, so that molecular biologists, and not ecologists or complexity biologist, have therefore been the ones receiving most of the funds and recognition.

Nowadays, biologists are beginning to shift their attention to genetic structures of epigenetic and metabolic networks, but we still know very little about the complex dynamics of these networks. Predictably, GMOs will lead to a decrease in biodiversity, and the loss of complexity within the environment will have detrimental effects on ecological equilibrium, likely endangering many more plant and animal species than those directly affected by the GMO's take-over of habitat.

Today, the people fighting to protect the environment must wage their battles against GMOs with scientists upholding the principles of genetic determinism. The latter are recognized and honored and given a voice in the media to guarantee the harmlessness of GMOs. Luckily, some people within medical and scientific institutes are starting to make themselves heard on the dangers of GMOs. In 1999, a contributor to *The Lancet* wrote:

> The issue of genetically modified foods has been badly mishandled by everyone involved. Governments should never have allowed these products into the food chain without insisting on rigorous testing for effects on health. The companies should have paid greater attention to the possible risks to health and of the public's perception of this risk; they are now paying the price of this neglect.[9]

Most of the adverse effects on the environment and human health will appear in the long term, so unfortunately they cannot be detected any time soon. The short-term effects that are presently visible, however, are the result of gene manipulation in animals—for example, to create fast-growing "supersalmon." There have also been cases in which genes have been extracted from fruit flies and inserted into mice, resulting in multiple and severe malformations in the mice, among them cerebral aplasia. Why anyone would make an animal suffer just to conduct these experiments is beyond me. Animals, just like plants, should be left to live in peace, as nature intends them to. It is wrong to try to speed up evolution at all costs. In its wisdom, nature has never produced monsters, yet man, with his intelligence, runs the risk of doing so. This reckless behavior has already resulted in numerous disasters. The ecological damage our planet has suffered stands as a testament to this. Calculations based on experimental evidence will have scientists underestimate the effects their tampering has on the environment and human health only to realize, often when it is too late, that the disasters that ensue are fatal. Throughout history many such disasters have occurred in the name of science or industry.

I have first-hand experience with the problems relating to occupational medicine. In countless cases workers have been exposed to substances initially thought to be harmless, and later discovered to be dangerous. A case in point is asbestos, on which I started my studies in Trieste. Asbestos is an inert substance, and for this reason it was initially thought to be harmless. So, for roughly ninety years, millions of workers were exposed to asbestos without knowing it was cancerous.

As I noted at the beginning of this book, many negative effects from exposure to carcinogens appear only after a long period of time, and sadly in the meantime many people continue to be exposed. Tragically, even long after it was proven that asbestos causes cancer, many workers continued to be exposed because of the scientific debates led by certain "scientists" who doubted the cancer-causing effect of the substance. Many workers have been exposed to concentrations of other substances that, like asbestos, were initially thought to be harmless. But the risks don't end here.

It is widely known that indiscriminate and reckless emissions of dangerous substances into the environment cause harm to human health and nature. I have personally battled for many toxic substances to be eliminated from the workplace, and as a member of the National Board of WWF Italy (World Wildlife Fund), I, together with my friends at WWF Italy, have waged an uphill battle in fighting the greenhouse effect and global warming.

In its thirty-plus years of activity, WWF has been reporting the global warming risks deriving from the rise in CO_2 levels and other pollutants in the atmosphere. Many so-called climate experts continued to deny this possibility, accusing public opinion of catastrophism. Now, as the effects of global warming are becoming blatantly obvious, no scientist in his right mind would dream of denying this reality. And yet, a handful of scientists, like the soldier who wouldn't quit, still continue to deny the facts and, although they admit that global warming exists, they attribute it to natural causes.

We cannot afford to be less than critical of modernity and its claims of progress, and we must reassess the blind trust we have placed in science and technology. No doubt science and technology have led us to enormous advancements, but we must acknowledge their dangerous potential, especially when we observe science's presumption in considering itself able to single-handedly manage the complexity of reality. Unlimited trust in reason and science to solve man's problems is one of the main reasons for the illnesses of modern Western society and culture. If Enlightenment gave rise to human, civil, and social progress and broke down social barriers, creating unprecedented social mobility through democracy and scientific development, the rationalism, positivism, and reductionism that ensued have led to the impoverishment of humans, reducing us to a mere instrument of rationality in the process of development. We have lost the features that so deeply characterized man in the age of Renaissance and later in the age of Enlightenment in his striving for harmonious and global development, only to be left, in the reductionism and "techno obsession" of this era, with cold and calculated reason.

Unless it is arrested in time, rationalism is driving man toward a dangerous anthropological mutation. The signs are crystal clear. Everything is measured exclusively in terms of growth. This is true in all fields, not just economic and financial arenas. It does not matter what you produce, as long as you produce more products—be they GMOs, or dangerous medicines of dubious benefit, or pollutants. Everything is consumed, becomes waste, and is thrown away. No doubt this is useful from an economic standpoint.

Our need to consume is reflected also in the vast quantities of land being exploited to build up and expand our ever-widening towns and cities in a mad race toward indiscriminate development led by politicians and architects, who are perpetrating enormous damage to humanity. Urban sprawl is in fact one of the main causes of environmental damage, contributing to the greenhouse effect and causing permanent soil and groundwater alteration (indeed, concreted land is unable to regain its natural characteristics for many decades, even after the buildings have been demolished).

Financially speaking, if a transaction leaves thousands of investors penniless but is lucrative for stakeholders, they won't think twice about it. The cold operation of capitalism whose only objective is to maximize profits is widening the gap between the haves and have-nots, creating severe social imbalance. The managing directors of large banks or companies guarantee profits to stakeholders and earn salaries that are unthinkable for the middle or lower-middle classes.

Today, the middle class is living the uncertainty of the future, for in this "liquid modernity," as Zygmunt Bauman calls it, our life is on a wire edge. It doesn't take much: unemployment or an illness and a person is suddenly in freefall. Cold rationality devoid of sensibility and willingness is leading us toward the loss of meaning. The enigma that is our life, which to be lived forces us to face an unavoidable question of meaning, today is nearly devoid of meaning. Everything has a price tag. You can sell your body, and also your soul. In the rat race, each person tries to survive and scratch out a living as best as he can.

The media sets absurd standards for life: beauty, success, power, money. If you have these things, you have it all, except the meaning of life and maybe the true joy. The loss of meaning is the feature that most characterizes the modern age. Never before has a society lacked so much meaning. You see it every day and can sense it in the air.

Cancer is one of the by-products of this loss of meaning. Cancer, as I said earlier, is a pathology of signification: the codes needed to communicate in living beings are changed in tumor pathologies. These codes attempt to reorganize and re-establish life in instances where it has lost meaning. Healing cancer also means finding meaning in our existence.

In these difficult times, I think the only path pursuable is within ourselves, in our profound self. We must tap into our inner strength to fight our egotistical instincts and have faith that something has meaning, regardless of the results achieved. It is not like fighting a windmill, but it may be the only way to stay alive in an atomized world where there is no longer a sense of community and in which an increasingly discretional and arbitrary power rises as the symbol of death.

We must help ourselves to understand that to save the world from imminent disaster we need specific virtues. Every age in history, as Ervin Laszlo reminds us, requires typical virtues to solve the specific problems of that era. Today the main virtue required of us, as again Laszlo points out,[10] is the sense of ecological responsibility—in other words, respect for our environment and other living beings. To save ourselves we need to ensure that the general interest is compatible with our own individual interest. The extreme individualism and egotism that characterizes our era has become incompatible with our survival. It is obscene for a few to waste the planet's resources, while the rest of the humanity lives in destitution and poverty, and "mere" plants and animals are crowded out entirely. Happiness does not exist if it is surrounded by suffering and unhappiness. Egotism and stupidity will have to confront a question of meaning: our existence is a brief journey through space and time and simply a tiny dot.

Seen from this perspective, we should be amazed at how much time and energy we waste chasing mirages. Life presents us at all times with an unavoidable request, the source of our anxiety and fear: "Find meaning." Today we are getting farther and farther away from answering this question. But we cannot avoid giving an answer, on pain of the loss of life itself. Today the ongoing assault on the planet evidences aspects of death. The obliteration of the blue sky in many metropolitan areas due to air pollution is a symbol of death. A society that obliterates its own sky is destined for extinction. Cancer is linked to growing pollution levels and is one result of this process that leads to death.

To retrieve meaning we must return to the roots of life. We come from the stars *(de-sidera),* in other words, from the primordial nucleus of matter that was formed at the origin of the universe. Our deepest desires *(desidera)* are linked to the universe through knowledge, the essence of our being and of the world. Knowing is in fact the act that, as Rudolf Steiner stated, reunites us with the world. Knowledge allows us to understand that we are part of the world and that if we respect all living beings and the world then we will respect ourselves and our lives. When we hurt others and hurt the environment, we hurt ourselves. We belong to the world and must reclaim our sense of belonging in order to widen our consciousness and give meaning to our existence, thereby conquering death.

This appendix analyzes in further detail the processes set out in Chapter 6 through which the fertilized egg becomes a complete being or, in other words, through which an embryo develops.

Embryo Development

During embryo development, cell multiplication and differentiation (or specialization) processes occur through a series of complex stages that take place at mind-boggling speed.

First, the stages regarding the replication process must be examined. These normally include a) the replication of genetic material within the cellular nucleus; b) the condensation and distribution of duplicated genetic material in each of the two daughter cells (segregation); and c) division of the cytoplasm and formation of all the organs the cytoplasmic membranes. The process in which cells divide to create two daughter cells that are genetically identical to the cell that generated them is called mitosis and occurs in somatic cells (body cells), while the process where cells halve the amount of genetic material and give rise to genetically different cells is called meiosis. This latter process forms germ cells and is at the basis of genetic variability, re-mixing hereditary material and producing new gene combinations. This process plays a fundamental role in sexual biological cycles. The phase when the cell is not dividing is the so-called interphase.

The Cellular Cycle

Cells are characterized by a two-phase cellular cycle: interphase and mitosis or, in the case of germ cells, meiosis. The interphase in turn can be divided into three sub-phases: G1, S, and G2. The cell duplicates its own genetic material during the S phase (synthesis). The period between the end of mitosis and the start of the S phase is known as G1 (the first gap). The second gap (G2) separates the end of the S phase and the start of mitosis, when nuclear and cytoplasmic division take place and two new cells are formed. Mitosis and cytoplasmic division are together indicated as the M phase of the cellular cycle. Even if the S phase occurs only through the replication of genetic material, fundamental processes of the cellular cycle also occur in the G1 and G2 phases. In the G1 phase, the cell prepares to enter into the S phase, with the "decision" to start a new cellular cycle made when the cell moves from the G1 phase to the S phase. During the G2 phase the cell finishes preparing itself for mitosis by, for example, synthesizing the microtubules that will move the chromosomes toward opposite poles of the cell during division.

The stimuli for genetic replication are generally chemical in nature. The embryo contains many such stimuli, known as growth factors. These act similarly within the microenvironment. They link up to the respective target proteins thanks to complex special receptors located on the surface of the cell. The link triggers specific events within the target cell that start a new cellular cycle. Within the cell, endogen control in the various phases of the cellular cycle is carried out by certain protein complexes called cyclin-dependent kinase. In addition to these complexes, other proteins are important to control the cell cycle. Among these are the pRb protein of the retinoblastoma (defined on the basis of an infantile neoplasia in which the protein was first identified), which controls the point of restriction halfway through the G1 phase and after which one cell irrevocably continues the rest of the cellular cycle. When the protein is not phosphorylated it blocks the cellular cycle, but when it is phosphorylated by cyclin-dependent kinase it stops blocking the point of restriction, thereby allowing the cell to move out of the G1 phase and into the S phase.

It is worth noting that cellular function occurs because an inhibitor, such as the retinoblastoma protein, has been inhibited in turn by a small modification occurring after the protein has synthesized, in this case by a phosphorylation process. This is a fairly common phenomenon in metabolism control and cell life processes.

Later in the text we will see this phenomenon appear again in the mechanisms that cause programmed cellular death in which, like two sides of a coin, some molecules are intent on self-destruction while others are focused on survival. Along with the pRb protein, the p53 protein is critical for cycle control. If DNA is damaged, this protein steps in by synthesizing the p21 protein, so-called because of its 21 kDaltons molecular weight. The p21 protein inhibits the kinase from being activated during the G1 phase and thereby stops the cellular cycle so that the cell can repair the damage. After the DNA has been repaired, the p21 protein is degraded, allowing the cyclin-dependent kinase to resume its function and continue the cellular cycle.

As we saw in cancer, the differentiation factors regulate the functions of the retinoblastoma and p53 proteins and stop the cell cycle of tumor cells. In this way mutations that are at the source of malignancies are repaired and the cells re-differentiate, as evidenced by the increase in differentiation markers such as E-caderin. However, when genetic damage cannot be repaired, programmed cellular death is activated and the cells die. It is widely known that mutations are the alteration of genetic material, usually DNA.

The Genetic Code

A gene is a segment of DNA that, as we will see later on, codifies the production of a polypeptide chain (protein) and contains the hereditary information of an organism. Genes are responsible for transmitting the hereditary traits that appear in each organism (phenotype).

Normally, each of us has various phenotypic traits, such as eye and hair color, facial and body features, etc., based on the genotype of which each one of us is made up. DNA, among the most famous icons of the twentieth century, replicates itself in a precise manner during the cellular division cycle.

DNA is made up of two strands that replicate in a semi-conservative way. Each strand acts as a mold for the synthesis of a new complementary strand. In this way, each of the two strands produced by the replication of a DNA molecule is made up of one parent strand and one newly synthesized strand.

The molecular make-up that replicates DNA is extremely complex and makes a mistake every million nucleotides added. (Nucleotides are the building blocks of DNA and are composed of sugar, deoxyribose, a phosphate group, and one of the following bases: adenine, guanine, thymine, and cytosine.) The bases in the double helix are dislocated so that adenine is always coupled with thymine and cytosine with guanine. As the two strands are complementary, if you know the nucleotidic sequence of one, it is possible to know that of the other.

When DNA mutates it is repaired through three different mechanisms: a) proofreading, whereby replication errors are corrected as they are made; b) mismatch reparation in which neo-synthesized DNA is scanned and then the errors are corrected; and c) split-off reparation in which the damaged pieces are separated from the rest.

In less complex organisms, such as germs (prokaryotes), DNA is a single long molecule bound to proteins, whereas in more complex organisms (eukaryotes), DNA is contained in discrete bodies called chromosomes visible during cell division. The number of chromosomes of an organism varies according to its species (the human species has forty-six chromosomes).

DNA is associated with a group of proteins called histones. During the interphase the chromosomes are packed into a dense structure called chromatin, which is contained in the nucleus and the rest of the nuclear membrane. In the process of cellular replication, the chromatin structure is loosened, enabling the DNA to duplicate and to copy in the corresponding RNA. RNA (ribonucleic acid) is similar to DNA in that it also is made up of a strand of nucleotides; however, it has a different sugar (ribose instead of deoxyribose) and base (uracil takes the place of thymine). Furthermore, unlike DNA molecules, RNA molecules are mostly composed of a single, shorter strand.

The process in which DNA is copied into RNA is known as transcription and involves only one of DNA's two strands. RNA undergoes a series of modifications; and lastly, messenger RNA (mRNA) is transported from the nucleus to the cytoplasm. Here it associates with a ribosome, a vast molecular complex made up of proteins and ribosomal RNA (rRNA).

After the transcription process, translation occurs. In mRNA nucleotides are organized into so-called "codons" of three bases that identify specific amino acids that join to form a polypeptide chain. For a specific amino acid, each codon codifies the building blocks that make up proteins. Alternatively, the codon functions as a starting or stopping point of translation of the polypeptide chain. The translation of the sequence of the RNA's nucleotides into amino acids of the polypeptide chain involves several enzymes and other molecules, among which are various types of a smaller form of RNA called transfer RNA (tRNA). These act as adapters by carrying the amino acids to the ribosome and adding them to the polypeptide chain being formed in the order dictated by the sequence of mRNA codons. All cell components are duplicated precisely so that the daughter cell is an exact copy of the mother cell.

This process takes place in the embryo during the first stages of development in which the fertilized egg multiplies without differentiating. Known as segmentation, this phase leads to the formation of the structure called a morula (berry) because of its shape, and the symmetrical division of the cells. Each mother cell divides into two identical daughter cells, as mentioned. These two cells become totipotent embryonic stem cells because, just like the fertilized egg, they can give rise to any kind of cell and therefore give life to a new being.

The Start of Cell Differentiation:
Various types of stem cells

As explained earlier, the segmentation phase is a multiplicative phase followed by a stage in which the first process of cellular differentiation begins. This process (and its embryonic structure) is called the blastocyst—an internal mass of cells that develops into an embryo from a hollow cavity surrounded by a layer of cells, which in mammals becomes the embryonic membrane and placenta.

In this stage not all embryonic cells are totipotent. Among the cells surrounding the blastocyst (on the outer layer), those that develop embryonic membranes start to differentiate. The totipotent cells of the internal mass of the blastocyst also start to differentiate into daughter cells, which give rise to three primary germ cell layers: ectoderm (which will develop into the skin, including mammary tissue and the nervous system), endoderm (which will develop into the tissue of the digestive system, including the digestive glands), and mesoderm (which will develop into bones, muscle, connective tissue, and blood vessels). The cell's loss of totipotency and gain of specialized functions is the consequence of an asymmetrical division (the mother cells on the one hand spawn identical daughter cells and on the other differing cells that have begun to differentiate). Subsequent divisions will create various types of stem cells which, according to their degree of specialization, will be defined as: a) pluripotent; b) multipotent; c) oligopotent; d) definitively differentiating cells; or e) completely differentiated cells. It should be pointed out that these cells gradually acquire specialized functions and progressively lose their ability to multiply. Indeed, completely differentiated cells are no longer able to multiply. Cells that in certain tissue of adult organisms continue to multiply and then differentiate such as bone marrow cells, cells that develop into blood cells, skin germ cells, or intestinal villus cells are in fact stem cells that remain in an adult organism.

How does differentiation occur from a totipotent parent cell? What are the underlying mechanisms? The progress made in molecular biology, the sequencing and understanding of genetic codes—though only part of the mechanisms that regulate gene expression—has led us to understand how a completely undifferentiated totipotent cell multiplying rapidly can become a specialized cell that is stable in replication terms.

At this point we must follow the chain of events through which information is exchanged among cells. In brief, the heart of the problem is understanding how this information is transmitted during replication/differentiation processes, making it possible for the genetic code, which is the same in all the cells of the organism, to carry out different functions in each specialized cell. Many of the advancements in knowledge, which I will now illustrate, have been made possible by the sequencing of the genetic code.

This fundamental step for biology aimed to unveil the deepest secrets of cellular functioning and reveal, as some have declared with no small amount of rhetoric and pomposity, the language of God in the creation of life. In actual fact this research undertaking made us realize, as often happens when important scientific goals have been achieved, that we are only beginning to understand how life is organized. Indeed, this is what makes science so fascinating. When you reach an objective that you think can take you to the next level in understanding a problem, you discover a world that is even vaster and more complex.

At this point, you must go back to the drawing board and try to comprehend ever greater levels of complexity. DNA sequencing served to help us understand many fascinating aspects of biology, such as:

A. In the human species less than two percent of the genetic code, totaling roughly 21,000 genes, is needed to codify proteins. Before the start of the sequencing process, it was estimated that there were between 80,000 and 100,000 codifying human genes. Such a low number of genes (in fact only slightly higher than that of the fruit fly) goes to show that the diversity observed in the protein molecules (which in humans number approximately 100,000) is the result of different regulation processes of single genes. In more complex organisms, such as humans, greater complexity is associated with a higher regulation capacity, instead of a higher quantity of codifying genes. A medium-sized eukaryotic gene in reality codifies more than a protein molecule. There are genes in certain eukaryotic organisms that codify more than 3,000 different proteins.

B. Genes vary greatly in size, from 1,000 to 2.4 million nucleotides.

C. Most (99.9%) of the human genome is identical in each member of a species. However, despite this apparent homogeny, there are many differences between individuals. More than two million differences have been mapped among single nucleotides.

D. Genes are not uniformly distributed in the genome. The 1 chromosome, with 2,968, is the highest, while the Y chromosome, which determines the male gender, is the lowest with 231.

E. More than fifty percent of the genome is made up of repetitive sequences. Much of the genome therefore does not serve to codify proteins. What then is the purpose of non-coding DNA? This type of DNA has long been referred to as "junk DNA." However, it has become increasingly clear that "junk DNA" instead has a function that is largely regulatory in nature. In other words, it regulates the same codifying genes as well as the signal mechanisms between cells.

The Epigenetic Code

It has clearly emerged that in addition to the genetic code, which is made up of genes that codify proteins, there is also a tight-knit network of molecules and a substantial portion of DNA that performs regulatory functions. Together the network and the regulating DNA make up the "epigenetic code." In reality it is a code that informs the precise system of regulation of gene expression during embryonic development, thereby determining which genes remain active and which ones do not; which protein products should be synthesized and which should not; which molecular communication mechanisms should remain operational and which should not; and in what way codifying genes should interact with their products. This is therefore the code that makes differentiation and specialization possible as the embryo develops. This is the code that enables a totipotent embryonic stem cell to become a liver cell, kidney cell, brain cell, lung cell, etc. Just as the conductor of an orchestra decides how a piece of music is to be played, so the epigenetic code decides how the codifying DNA within each cell should be read. In this way, when the differentiation process has been completed, all the differentiated cells have the same DNA as their base, but the part of active codifying genes in each differently specialized cell is specifically different and represents only a fraction of the entire DNA that it is able to codify. With the exception of a very few cases, the differences between specialized cells are epigenetic and not genetic. Today the study of epigenetics is changing the face of biology. The twenty-first century starts as the century of epigenetics, shifting the spotlight that was until now directed solely on the genetic code.

We still do not realize the extent of these changes, even if the prospects for the future in the therapeutic field are likely to stem from this branch of research rather than from genetics, where results linked to genetic manipulation have been disappointing and ethically questionable.

Let us at this point examine the various stages of epigenetic regulation to which totipotent embryonic stem cells are subject until they become fully differentiated cells. As I already mentioned, in a multicellular organism with specialized cells and tissue, each cell possesses all the genes of that organism. The difference between specialized cells is due to the specific activity of the genes that continue to function even after the specific and selective silencing to which many of them are subject during the differentiation of the embryonic cell. For the development to continue normally and for each cell to acquire and maintain a specialized function, certain proteins must therefore be synthesized at the right moment and in the right cell. Therefore, gene expression must be controlled in a very precise manner. Unlike DNA replication, which generally in each cell is regulated according to the "all or nothing" principle, gene expression is a highly selective process.

Chromatin Remodeling

One of the first places in which the regulatory process occurs is at the chromatin level, which, as mentioned, is the material contained in the cell nucleus and is composed of dense DNA wrapped around a center made up of proteins called histones, which play an important role in compacting nucleic acid.

Two DNA folds, composed of 146 nucleotides, wrap around a center composed of eight histones to form a structure that resembles a pearl in a necklace—this is called a "nucleosoma." With the help of other histone proteins that link the centers of the various nucleosomes with the DNA interposed between them, the string of nucleosomes folds and becomes a chromatin fiber that is further compacted. The degree of chromatin density affects accessibility to important factors for the transcription of the genes contained therein. The more compact the chromatin, the less accessible the transcription factors. One way to keep a gene from transcribing is through methylation, whereby a group of CH_3 is attached to some of cells' bases. In this case the DNA sequence is not modified, but the chromatin is compacted, thereby determining the probability of transcription, which at this point is lower. Conversely, adding acetyl groups (C_2H_5) to certain amino acids of histones usually leads to a looser chromatin structure, thereby increasing the likelihood of transcription. Removing the acetylic groups from the histone proteins, like methylating their amino acids, renders the chromatin denser and does not allow the DNA to be transcribed. The remodeling of the chromatin can involve an entire chromosome—for example, one of the X chromosomes determining gender. It is widely known that normal female mammals have two X chromosomes while normal male mammals have an X chromosome and a Y chromosome. Between males and females there is a sizable difference in terms of the "dosage" of genes linked to the X chromosome. In other words, each cell of a female has two copies of genes present in the X chromosome and can potentially produce twice the proteins codified by these genes compared to male cells. This does not occur because during cell differentiation one of the two maternal X chromosomes is methylated and its chromatin condensed in such a way that the DNA sequences become inaccessible to the molecular transcription machinery.

Transcriptional and Post-Transcriptional Regulation

This highly complex machinery is made up of proteins called transcription factors that are necessary for an enzyme called RNA polymerases to form a complex that determines the starting point of transcription. This complex binds to a DNA sequence called a promoter and is where the transcription of the codifying region of the gene is promoted. At the opposite end of this latter is a region of the DNA called terminator, the point at which transcription is terminated. In this way start and stop signals occur in the transcription of DNA into RNA.

At transcriptional level there are many regulatory events that significantly change gene expression. Regulating regions have been recently discovered that are immediately grouped at the origin of the promoter. Various regulating proteins can link up to these regions and can activate transcription. Far from the promoter, even 20,000 bases away, we find intensifying sequences (intensifiers). These sequences bind activating proteins, greatly stimulating the transcription complex. Lastly, in DNA there are negative regulating regions called silencing sequences that have the opposite effect of intensifiers. Silencers arrest transcription and link proteins aptly call suppressors. In some cases gene expression is regulated by the movement of a gene to a new position on the chromosome, and as a result the DNA is rearranged. This rearrangement is important, among other things, for producing highly variable proteins, such as those that make up the repertoire of human antibodies. Rearrangement is also important in determining certain forms of cancer in which inactive genes can seem to have moved next to active promoters.

Another type of regulation is known as genetic amplification. This occurs, for example, in the mature egg cells of frogs and fish. After fertilization, a trillion ribosomes are necessary for protein synthesis. Cells that differentiate into egg cells initially contain less than one thousand copies of genes that codify for the ribosomal RNA. It would take about fifty years to synthesize that much RNA. Egg cells have solved this problem by selectively increasing the group of genes for ribosomal RNA, thereby hugely increasing the quantity. In fact, this group of genes rises from 0.2% to 68% of total codifying DNA. These million copies that transcribe very quickly synthesize in just a few days the trillion ribosomes needed for the next protein synthesis.

In terms of post-transcriptional regulation processes, I must point out that an extremely important mechanism in superior organisms is linked to a process known as "alternative RNA splicing." In the DNA of eukaryotes, codifying sequences called exons are next to non-codifying sequences, known as introns. Transcribed introns appear in the primary RNA transcriptions called pre mRNA which, before arriving in the cytoplasm of the ribosomes, undergo a splicing process that occurs in large complexes of RNA and proteins called "spliceosomes." In this splicing process the introns of primary transcription of the RNA are eliminated, and the exons are grouped together. This messenger RNA (mature mRNA) is translated into polypeptides (proteins). Splicing is often very complex, as it can make many different cuts that are able to give rise to multiple messenger RNA and consequently to differing protein products. (For example, in *Drosophila melanogaster* this process leads to the synthesis of up to three thousand different proteins.) Another post-transcriptional regulatory event is the one linked to RNA editing, which takes place essentially either by inserting new nucleotides into the mRNA or by chemically modifying a nucleotide. In both cases the synthesized protein is modified. Even the survival time of messenger RNA in the cytoplasm undergoes post-transcriptional regulation. The less time mRNA spends in the cytoplasm, the fewer the codified proteins synthesized by mRNA.

Finally, regulation mechanisms that are important in terms of transcription and post-transcriptions—and also, as we will see, in terms of translation—are those linked to the action of RNA regulators. (Scientists are discovering that RNA makes up numerous and large families, and as research develops the functions of these families are gaining greater importance.) These RNAs were basically discovered after failed attempts on the part of researchers to obtain new functions or modifications in plants and animals by inserting in their cells fragments of DNA or RNA. For example, by introducing an extra copy of the gene that develops into the color magenta in petunias, researchers hoped to obtain more colorful flowers. Instead, they wound up with white flowers or white and magenta flowers. This meant that the new gene introduced and the plant's pre-existing genes had in some way deactivated. Similar examples of genetic silencing have been found in fungi and animals.

For a while these anomalies were the object of discussions, referred to from time to time as "suppressors" in plants, "suffocators" in fungi, and "interfering RNA" in animals. Researchers finally acknowledged that these share common elements. Now they are collectively known as interfering RNA. Interfering RNA leads to genetic silencing and is dependent on small RNA molecules called siRNA (small interfering RNAs) that derive from larger RNA molecules with an unusual structure. These molecules are double stranded and are recognized by an enzyme called "Dicer" that reduces the molecules into small "dice" measuring from 21 to 23 nucleotides in length. These RNA molecules are able to cause the destruction of copies of aberrant messenger RNA, from which they derive, and associate themselves with the complementary sequences present in mRNA and therefore induce another enzyme to destroy it. Any messenger RNA with sequences that are complementary to these small RNAs undergoes the same process. As a result, the gene responsible for the transcription of the messenger RNA does not express itself.

Another bizarre trait of these small RNAs is their ability to move to other cells, even different types, and thus cause genetic silencing from a distance. They are also able to silence genes through the stable methylation of DNA, as mentioned earlier. In this case, regulation is at transcriptional level. The Dicer enzyme frees another class of small RNA starting from a double-stranded precursor. These molecules are processed by the Dicer and end up being reduced to single-stranded molecules measuring from 21 to 23 nucleotides in length. These are known as micro RNA (miRNA), and they recognize the sequence of target messenger RNAs and mate with them, thereby keeping the latter from being translated into proteins. In this case the action mechanism is different. We can speak of translational regulation, a mechanism that we will address later and not a post-transcriptional regulation mechanism, which leads to the destruction of messenger RNA. MiRNA is involved in cell differentiation and has a significant impact on the regulation of gene expression and therefore on the development of an organism. Studies in which a part of the machinery of miRNA processing was destroyed have shown that an organism cannot survive without the regulator role that miRNA plays. Through interfering RNA it is possible to virtually deactivate in a selective manner any gene simply by introducing a miRNA inside a cell. The potential benefits arising from the application of this technique are enormous.

Translational and Post-Translational Regulation

Having addressed how specific microRNA uses the translation regulation mechanism to block the translation of specific mRNA (which obviously prevents the corresponding proteins from being synthesized), I will now focus on translation regulation events. These latter are often connected to the concentration of specific proteins that need to be synthesized. When their concentration is low, the speed at which messenger RNA already present in the cytoplasm translates them increases. Inversely, when their concentration is high, translation slows down. Lastly, proteins can be regulated after they have been synthesized. An important post-translation regulation event is tied to the control of survival time of proteins within the cell itself. We have seen how some proteins involved in cellular division, like cyclins, are hydrolyzed at just the right moment so that sequencing can develop correctly over time. In many instances a protein that is to be degraded is linked to a polypeptide chain composed of 76 amino acids called ubiquitin (so-called because it is ubiquitous). This complex in turn binds to another large complex made up of a dozen polypeptides called proteasomes, which compose a sort of molecular destruction chamber in which the degrading protein is destroyed. The fact that so many proteins are concentrated within the cell is not determined by the differing speeds of transcription of the genes, but rather by how fast proteasomes destroy the molecules.

Another example of a protein undergoing post-translational regulation—which has nothing to do with embryonic differentiation but addressed here for the sake of completeness—is the infamous "mad cow" syndrome (bovine spongiform encephalopathy or BSE). This is an obvious example of a pathology of post-translational regulation. Many proteins, as occurs in many other macromolecules, can take on different forms depending on the context, even though they maintain the same amino acid sequence. These differing protein conformations ("conformational landscapes") often have different functions. BSE arises from the presence of a protein in a non-functioning form that in its normal form is key to brain health. BSE is caused by the same pathological protein codified by the non-mutated corresponding gene, which, after having been translated, takes on an anomalous conformation. The non-functioning protein invades the brain cells, which end up dying.

The formation process of an anomalous protein is highly unique. A normally conformed protein becomes anomalous when it meets an anomalous protein. The anomalous protein mates with the normal protein and changes its conformation: a classic example of a bad influence. The disease then spreads within the nervous system and the individual eventually dies. The disease is transferred from one organism to another by eating meat in which cells in the nervous system contain anomalous proteins. These proteins behave as described above and cause the disease. All the gene regulation processes that we have examined, except this last one, are responsible for differentiating events that occur in the embryo and therefore for the processes that make a totipotent fertilized egg cell become a whole organism.

In short, I have analyzed how cellular differentiation consists of a differential, specific, and selective gene regulation process that essentially restricts the expressed genome. A cell's gene expression after each stage of differentiation varies from the progenitor cell in terms of hundreds of expressed genes. This is possible, as I mentioned earlier, because a gene, which in the past was thought to be the control center independent and autonomous from protein synthesis, in actual fact is directly and indirectly controlled by a regulation network and by synthesized proteins. In the embryo the intense and extended interaction between the nucleus and the cytoplasm and the cytoplasm and the microenvironment is a prime example of complexity. An embryo under development and differentiation is indeed an excellent example of what complexity researchers have coined the "complex adaptive system."

Composed of a network of multiple cells that act in parallel and have differing levels of organization that are constantly under revision and control, this system has an implicit prediction written in the genetic code and in the epigenetic regulatory events. The system is in continuous transition and changes constantly emerge. In this way, the totipotent stem cells (parent cells of all other cells) first give rise to pluripotent stem cells, then multipotent stem cells, and then oligopotent cells, and so on until a new being is formed.

Table of Known Human Carcinogens

Overall Evaluations of Carcinogenicity to Humans
Group 1: Carcinogenic to humans

As evaluated in *IARC Monographs* Volumes 1–98
This list contains all agents evaluated as being in Group 1 to date.

Group 1: *Carcinogenic to humans* (102)
Agents and groups of agents

4-Aminobiphenyl
Arsenic
Asbestos
Azathioprine
Benzene
Benzidine
Benzo[*a*]pyrene
Beryllium
N,N-Bis(2-chloroethyl)-2-naphthylamine (Chlornaphazine)
Bis(chloromethyl)ether and chloromethyl methyl ether
1,3-Butadiene
1,4-Butanediol dimethanesulfonate (Busulphan; Myleran)
Cadmium
Chlorambucil
1-(2-Chloroethyl)-3-(4-methylcyclohexyl)-1-nitrosourea
    (Methyl-CCNU; Semustine)
Chromium
Ciclosporin
Cyclophosphamide
Diethylstilboestrol
Epstein-Barr virus

Erionite

Estrogen-progestogen menopausal therapy (combined)

Estrogen-progestogen oral contraceptives (combined)

(NB: There is also convincing evidence in humans that these agents confer a protective effect against cancer in the endometrium and ovary)

Estrogens, nonsteroidal

(NB: This evaluation applies to the group of compounds as a whole and not necessarily to all individual compounds within the group)

Estrogens, steroidal (NB: This evaluation applies to the group of compounds as a whole and not necessarily to all individual compounds within the group)

Estrogen therapy, postmenopausal

Ethanol in alcoholic beverages

Ethylene oxide

Etoposide in combination with cisplatin and bleomycin

Formaldehyde

Gallium arsenide

Gamma Radiation: see X- and Gamma (g)-Radiation

Helicobacter pylori (infection with)

Hepatitis B virus (chronic infection with)

Hepatitis C virus (chronic infection with)

Human immunodeficiency virus type 1 (infection with)

Human papillomavirus types 16, 18, 31, 33, 35, 39, 45, 51, 52, 56, 58, 59 and 66 (NB: The HPV types that have been classi fied as *carcinogenic to humans* can differ by an order of magnitude in risk for cervical cancer)

Human T-cell lymphotropic virus type I

Melphalan

8-Methoxypsoralen (Methoxsalen plus ultraviolet A radiation) MOPP and other combined chemotherapy including alkylating agents

Mustard gas (Sulfur mustard)

2-Naphthylamine

Neutrons

(NB: Overall evaluation upgraded from 2B to 1 with supporting
evidence from other relevant data)

Nickel compounds

N'-Nitrosonornicotine (NNN) and 4-(N-Nitrosomethylamino)-
1-(3-pyridyl)-1-butanone (NNK)

[Oestrogen: see Estrogen]

Opisthorchis viverrini (infection with)

Oral contraceptives, combined estrogen-progestogen: see
Estrogen-progestogen oral contraceptives (combined)

Oral contraceptives, sequential

Phosphorus-32, as phosphate

Plutonium-239 and its decay products (may contain plutonium-
240 and other isotopes), as aerosols

Radioiodines, short-lived isotopes, including iodine-131, from
atomic reactor accidents and nuclear weapons detonation
(exposure during childhood)

Radionuclides, a-particle-emitting, internally deposited

(NB: Specific radionuclides for which there is *sufficient* evidence
for carcinogenicity to humans are also listed individually as
Group 1 agents)

Radionuclides, b-particle-emitting, internally deposited

(NB: Specific radionuclides for which there is *sufficient* evidence
for carcinogenicity to humans are also listed individually as
Group 1 agents)

Radium-224 and its decay products

Radium-226 and its decay products

Radium-228 and its decay products

Radon-222 and its decay products

Schistosoma haematobium (infection with)

Silica crystalline (inhaled in the form of quartz or cristobalite from occupational sources)

Solar radiation

Talc containing asbestiform fibres

Tamoxifen

(NB: There is also conclusive evidence that tamoxifen reduces the
   risk of contralateral breast cancer)

2,3,7,8-Tetrachlorodibenzo-*para*-dioxin

(NB: Overall evaluation upgraded from 2A to 1 with supporting
   evidence from other relevant data)

Thiotepa

Thorium-232 and its decay products, administered intravenously
   as a colloidal dispersion of thorium-232 dioxide

Treosulfan

Vinyl chloride

X- and Gamma (g)-Radiation

Mixtures

Aflatoxins (naturally occurring mixtures of)

Alcoholic beverages

Areca nut

(NB: Overall evaluation based on human data, animal data, and
   mechanistic and other relevant data)

Betel quid with tobacco

Betel quid without tobacco

Coal-tar pitches

Coal-tars

Herbal remedies containing plant species of the genus
   Aristolochia

Household combustion of coal, indoor emissions from

Mineral oils, untreated and mildly treated

Phenacetin, analgesic mixtures containing

Salted fish (Chinese-style)

Shale-oils

Soots
Tobacco, smokeless
Wood dust

Exposure circumstances

Aluminium production
Arsenic in drinking-water
Auramine, manufacture of
Boot and shoe manufacture and repair
Chimney sweeping
Coal gasification
Coal-tar distillation
Coke production
Furniture and cabinet making
Haematite mining (underground) with exposure to radon
Involuntary smoking (exposure to secondhand or
    "environmental" tobacco smoke)
Iron and steel founding
Isopropyl alcohol manufacture (strong-acid process)
Magenta, manufacture of
Painter (occupational exposure as a)
Paving and roofing with coal-tar pitch
Rubber industry
Strong-inorganic-acid mists containing sulfuric acid
Tobacco smoking and tobacco smoke

Source: International Agency for Research on Cancer (IARC)
    Last updated: 29 November 2007

1. E.N. Lorenz, *Predictability: Does the flap of a butterfly's wings in Brazil set off a tornado in Texas?* Speech held at the American Association for Advancement of Science convention in Washington, DC, 29 December 1979.
2. *Osmizze* is the local word for eateries in the area of Trieste that during wine-making season attach grape leaves outside the restaurant as a sign to customers that *novello* wine is served.
3. Duncan Watts, *Reti di piccoli mondi in Complessità e Biologia,* edited by Pier Mario Biava (Milano, Italy: Bruno Mondadori, 2002).
4. Umberto Eco, *I limiti dell'interpretazione* (Milano, Italy: Bompiani, 1990), p. 222.
5. The term "code" has a different meaning depending on the discipline being referred to. "Semiotics [...] defines a code as a system of signification that associates entities that are present and perceptible to the senses to absent entities through a body of rules correlational between codifying systems (expression) and codified systems (content). Theoreticians of communication instead view 'code' as a system that enables information to be transmitted and filed and that is composed of a group of signals (the alphabet) and a system of rules (grammar)." M.A. Villamira, *Comunicazione e Interazione. Aspetti del comportamento interpersonale e sociale* (Milano, Italy: Franco Angeli, 1997).

   In linguistics, codes are corresponding systems between the order of expression and the order of content that serve to transmit information between a sender and a receiver by making and issuing messages. In semiotics, a code is a necessary preliminary condition for signification. The fact that the receiver receives the message and the receiver's interpretative behavior are not necessary conditions for signification. "As long as the code establishes a link between the 'stands for' and the entity related thereto then the link can be useful for any possible recipient." M.A. Villamira, *ibid.*

From a semiotic perspective, therefore, the process of signification does not require an interpreter, but a code. In terms of codes, I point out how Umberto Eco wrote as early as 1984 on biological codes: "The start of a code is found in the S biological codes in which an object becomes significant because of the structure that is able to 'read' it. The reading establishes the code. The structure forms a sort of 'complementarity toward' the object set up embryonically as a sign. The code forms itself so obscurely at the basis of life like a story of choice, selection, sifting, sanctioned by the 'judge,' that is the complex of the things that storms or welcomes the complementarity that is established." Umberto Eco, *Semiotics and Philosophy of Language* (Turin, Italy: Einaudi, 1984).

In view of what we have said until now on the role of the epigenetic and genetic codes at embryonic level, the words of Eco seem almost prophetic.

6. Eva Jablonka and Marion J. Lamb, *Evolution in Four Dimensions: Genetic, Epigenetic, Behavioral, and Symbolic Variation in the History of Life* (Cambridge, MA: MIT Press, 2005).

7. Ervin Laszlo, *Science and the Akashic Field: An integral theory of everything* (Rochester, NY: Inner Traditions International, 2004).

8. Published in the *Sole 24ore,* 16 June 2007, page 10.

9. "Health risks of genetically modified foods." Editorial *Lancet* 353 (1999), p. 1811.

10. Ervin Laszlo, *Macroshift: Navigating the Transformation to a Sustainable World* (San Francisco: Berret Koehler Publishers, Inc., 2001). See also Ervin Laszlo, *The Chaos Point: The World at the Crossroads* (Charlottesville, VA: Hampton Roads, 2006).

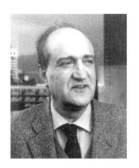

About the Author

Pier Mario Biava received his degree in medicine from the University of Pavia in 1969. He went on to specialize in occupational medicine at the University of Padova and in hygiene at the University of Trieste. Dr. Biava worked at the Institute of Occupational Medicine at the University of Trieste, where he taught Industrial Toxicology, Industrial Technology, and Epidemiology of Occupational Diseases. He has been studying environmental carcinogens since 1974.

Dr. Biava has performed numerous epidemiological studies, particularly about the relationship between asbestos and cancer, and has been studying the relationship between stem cell differentiation (when adult stem cells divide and create fully differentiated daughter cells during tissue repair and during normal cell turnover) and cancer since 1982. He was head of Occupational Medicine at the Hospital of Sesto S.G. (Milan), a professor at the Post-Graduate School of Occupational Medicine at the University of Trieste until 2001, and currently works at the Institute of Research and Cure of Scientific Character (IRCSC) Multimedica of Milan. Dr. Biava is the author of more than a hundred scientific publications and several books. He is vice president of the International Academy of Tumor Marker Oncology and a member of the editorial advisory boards of several scientific journals. In addition, Dr. Biava is president of the Foundation for Research into the Biological Therapies of Cancer and vice president of World Wildlife Fund Italy. He lives in Milan.